Dermatology

Robin Graham-Brown
BSc (Hons), MB BS (London), FRCP (London)
Consultant Dermatologist, University Hospitals of Leicester, UK and
Honorary Senior Lecturer in Dermatology, University of Leicester, UK
Editor of the British Journal of Dermatology 2001–2004
President-elect British Association of Dermatologists 2005–2006

John Savin
MA, MD (Cantab), FRCP (London and Edinburgh), DIH
Former President of the British Association of Dermatologists and of
the Dermatology Section of the Royal Society of Medicine, and
Consultant Dermatologist at The Royal Infirmary of Edinburgh, UK

Janeen Milner
BSc, MBChB, FRNZCGP, Dip Paeds, DFFP
General Practitioner, Leicester and Clinical Assistant in Dermatology,
Leicester Royal Infirmary, UK

CHURCHILL LIVINGSTONE

Edinburgh London New York Oxford Philadelphia St Louis Sydney Toronto 2004

Churchill Livingstone
An imprint of Elsevier Limited.

 is a registered trademark of Elsevier Limited.

ISBN 0443 074712

Cataloguing in Publication Data
Catalogue records for this book are available from the US Library of Congress and the British Library.

Note
Medical knowledge is constantly changing. As new information becomes available, changes in treatment, procedures, equipment and the use of drugs become necessary. The author and the publishers have taken care to ensure that the information given in this text is accurate and up to date. However, readers are strongly advised to confirm that the information, especially with regard to drug usage, complies with the latest legislation and standards of practice.

Printed in China

Contents

Preface   v

Biographies   vii

Acne   8

Actinic keratosis   15

Alopecia areata   17

Artefactual skin diseases   19

Basal cell carcinoma   21

Bowen's disease   23

Candidiasis   24

Dermatofibroma   25

Dermatophyte infections   27

Discoid lupus erythematosus   31

Eczema/dermatitis   33

Erysipelas   46

Head lice   48

Herpes simplex   51

Ichthyosis   54

Impetigo   56

Keratoacanthoma   58

Lichen planus   59

Lichen simplex   62

Melanocytic naevi   64

Melanoma (malignant)   66

Molluscum contagiosum   69

Painful nodule of the ear   72

Pemphigoid   73

Photosensitivity 75

Pityriasis versicolor 79

Pruritus (generalized) 81

Psoriasis 84

Pyogenic granuloma 90

Rosacea 91

Scabies 93

Seborrhoeic keratosis 97

Squamous cell carcinoma 98

Urticaria and angio-oedema 99

Vasculitis 105

Venous ulcers 108

Vitiligo 111

Warts (viral) 113

Case studies 119

Appendices 127

Index 165

Preface

Our selection of topics for *In Clinical Practice: Dermatology* has been dictated by simple mathematics. Given that there are 2000 skin conditions, fitting them all into 25,000 words would allow us only 13 words per subject – one sentence each perhaps, but not much more.

A more sensible set of sums could be based on the fact that 15% of consultations in general practice are for skin conditions, and that 70% of these fit into just nine types of skin disorder. Should we limit ourselves to these?

Again the balance seemed wrong. As a compromise, we have picked 40 conditions for this book. GPs will meet them all regularly.

Three other points are worth mentioning about this book. First, we have tried to make our treatment suggestions as "evidence based" as possible. However, a quick search of the Cochrane Library shows there are still huge gaps in the research on which such evidence can be based.

Second, while we have included some clinical photographs, this book is not meant to be an atlas of dermatology. There are enough of those already.

Finally, we have tried to avoid hiding behind polysyllabic dermatological terms. In the past these were a way of achieving what lawyers still call "the preservation of client ignorance." In other words, making a subject seem so difficult that only a specialist can possibly cope with it.

We hope that readers of this book will be find our guide to the "Top 40" skin conditions meets all these aims.

Robin Graham-Brown
Consultant Dermatologist, University Hospitals of Leicester, UK and Honorary Senior Lecturer in Dermatology, University of Leicester, UK
Editor of the British Journal of Dermatology 2001–2004
President-elect British Association of Dermatologists 2005–2006

John Savin
Former President of the British Association of Dermatologists and of the Dermatology Section of the Royal Society of Medicine, and Consultant Dermatologist at The Royal Infirmary of Edinburgh, UK

Janeen Milner
General Practitioner and Clinical Assistant in Dermatology
Leicester Royal Infirmary, UK

Biographies

Robin Graham-Brown BSc (Hons), MB BS (London), FRCP (London) graduated in medicine from the Royal Free Hospital School of Medicine, University of London, UK. His postgraduate training in general medicine and dermatology was also in London, at the Queen Mary's University Hospital and at the Royal Free. He was appointed Consultant Dermatologist in Leicester in 1983, and subsequently became Honorary Senior Lecturer in the university department.

His main clinical research interests have been in early diagnosis and public education on skin cancer (especially melanoma) and in atopic eczema.

Dr Graham-Brown has co-edited *Skin Diseases in the Elderly*, and co-written two books (*Lecture Notes on Dermatology* and *A Colour Atlas and Text of Dermatology*), as well as chapters for several textbooks. He has co-authored over 180 original articles, reviews and published abstracts.

John Savin MA, MD (Cantab), FRCP (London and Edinburgh), DIH has long been interested in the way dermatology impinges on general practice. He was Editor of the journal *Dermatology in Practice* from 1995 to 1999, and has co-written books on *Common Diseases of the Skin*, *Common Skin Problems* and on *Clinical Dermatology* (now in its third edition). He was also adviser in dermatology to the British Medical Association's *Complete Family Health Encyclopaedia* and *Complete Family Health Guide*.

Within dermatology, his main research interests have been in itching and scratching, epidemiology, bullous disorders and skin bacteriology.

Janeen Milner BSc, MBChB, FRNZCGP, Dip Paeds, DFFP is a Massey Scholar with a BSc in biochemistry. She completed her medical training at the University of Otago and has subsequently gained diplomas in paediatrics and family planning. Dr Milner trained in general practice and is a fellow of the New Zealand Royal College of General Practice.

Dr Milner is a New Zealander who has lived in the UK since 2001. She is a General Practitioner in an inner-city practice in Leicester and is Clinical Assistant in Dermatology at Leicester Royal Infirmary.

ACNE

Introduction and background

More people have acne than any other skin disorder and its appearance, however trivial it seems to others, often interferes with their enjoyment of life. Scarring perpetuates this. Treatment for acne must therefore be early and vigorous.[1]

Definition and epidemiology

> *Acne is a chronic inflammatory disorder of pilosebaceous follicles*

Acne is a chronic inflammatory disorder of pilosebaceous follicles. It is easy to identify as a mixture of the lesions shown in Figure 1 on a background of greasy skin (see Figure 2).

Acne affects the sexes equally in the teens and most adolescents have it. Thereafter it usually resolves slowly, although some 1% of men and 5% of women still have acne at age 40. The severity of acne in the population has declined over the last half century.

Aetiology

Several factors combine to cause acne.

Genetics

The high concordance rates for acne in identical twins and the frequent history of acne in the parents of patients suggest that genetic factors are important, but the mode of inheritance has not yet been established.

Hormonal

The high sebum excretion rate of most male acne patients is an excessive response of their sebaceous glands to normal androgen levels. The

Fig. 1. Types of lesions seen in acne.

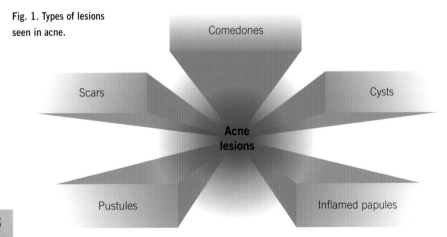

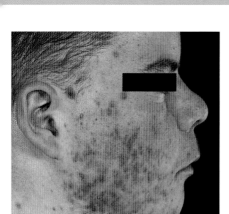

Fig. 2. Erythematous papules on the cheeks of a greasy skinned adolescent male. Reproduced with kind permission from Graham-Brown R and Bourke JF. Mosby's Colour Atlas and Text of Dermatology. London: Mosby Ltd, 1999.

picture is more complicated in females. Some may have an androgenic hormonal imbalance, for example caused by polycystic ovarian syndrome. Usually, however, the slight rise in free testosterone levels is due to low sex hormone binding globulin rather than to high testosterone.

Altered pattern of keratinization within the pilosebaceous follicles

This leads to comedones. Androgens play a part here too, as do environmental factors such as cosmetics.

Bacterial

Proprionobacterium acnes, a normal skin commensal, is present in large numbers in obstructed follicles and produces inflammatory mediators that diffuse into the surrounding tissue. The growing resistance of the organism to antibiotics, and particularly to erythromycin, may sometimes be responsible for lack of treatment success.

Diagnosis

The differential diagnosis is straightforward as only acne has the set of lesions mentioned earlier (see "Definition and epidemiology"), seen against a background of seborrhoea. If in doubt, consider the conditions listed in Figure 3.

Fig. 3. Conditions to consider before diagnosing acne.

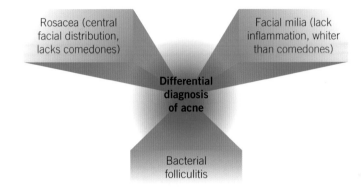

Rosacea (central facial distribution, lacks comedones)

Facial milia (lack inflammation, whiter than comedones)

Differential diagnosis of acne

Bacterial folliculitis

Fig. 4. Subtypes of acne.

Subtype	Example or features
Drug-induced acne	For example, from corticosteroids, androgens including anabolic steroids, phenytoin and isoniazid
Cosmetic acne	From greasy preparations Comedones are a prominent feature
Occupational acne	For example from oils, tars and chlorinated hydrocarbons
Mechanical acne	Due to pressure from objects such as violins
Infantile	Seen mainly in boys up to age 5
Late-onset acne	Stubborn and persistent Occurs in women more than men Usually seen on the chin
Excoriated acne	Usually seen in young girls The marks are the result of picking and digging at the skin True acne lesions may be minimal
Severe forms	Acne conglobata, which has deep nodules and sinuses Acne fulminans, which has an acute onset and is accompanied by fever and arthropathy

In addition, bear in mind that acne has several subtypes (Figure 4).

The diagnosis of acne is made clinically and investigations are seldom needed. Occasionally the following tests are worthwhile:

- Cultures to exclude bacterial folliculitis.
- If virilization is present, check circulating hormone levels and request ultrasound examination of adrenals and ovaries.
- Patients with the polycystic ovarian syndrome may have modestly elevated testosterone, androstenedione and dehydroepiandrosterone levels, a reduced sex hormone-binding level, and a luteinizing hormone to follicle stimulating hormone ratio greater than 2.5 to 1.

Prevention

Modifying the diet usually has little effect but many sufferers from acne avoid foods they think worsen their eruption. Gentle facial cleansing with soap and water or an antibacterial wash may help.

Treatment

General principles

The aims of treatment are shown in Figure 5.

Treatment should start early in the course of the disease, and be given with sympathy and encouragement, clear instructions and realistic expectations. Patients should always be told about possible side-effects.

Topical treatment

Figure 6 offers suggestions for treating mild acne. Topical corticosteroids should be avoided.

Physical treatments

These include:

- Incision and drainage of cysts.
- Dermabrasion, which may be used after acne has settled to smooth

66 Modifying the diet usually has little effect but many sufferers from acne avoid foods they think worsen their eruption 99

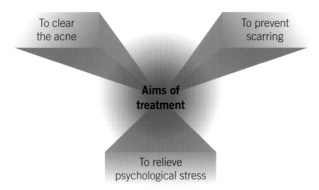

Fig. 5. The aims of treatment are threefold.

To clear the acne

To prevent scarring

Aims of treatment

To relieve psychological stress

Fig. 6. Topical treatments for mild acne.

Type of acne	Preparation	Notes
Mainly comedones	Topical retinoid or adapalene	Avoid exposure to the sun. Avoid during pregnancy. Women of childbearing age should take contraceptive precautions.
Comedones plus inflammation	Benzoyl peroxide	Start with lowest strength and increase gradually. Skin irritation at the start may subside with time. May bleach clothing and hair.
	Azaleic acid	Avoid during pregnancy and while breastfeeding. Less irritant than benzoyl peroxide.
Mainly inflammatory	A topical antibiotic such as clindamycin or erythromycin	If possible use topical antibacterial agents, such as benzoyl peroxide or azaleic acid, to avoid bacterial resistance. Also avoid using a topical antibiotic at the same time as a different systemic one. If repeated courses are needed, separate them by a short intervening course of a topical antibacterial agent.

scars, but it can lead to unsightly hyperpigmentation in dark skins. Skin resurfacing with lasers is now replacing this treatment.
- 8-week courses of ultraviolet irradiation, to help exacerbations.
- Cosmetic camouflage for scars.

66 Oral treatment is usually needed for moderate-to-severe acne, in conjunction with topical therapy 99

Oral treatment
This is usually needed for moderate-to-severe acne, in conjunction with topical therapy. The three main options are shown in Figure 7.

Antibiotics
The first choice is usually one of the tetracyclines, preferably oxytetra-cycline or tetracycline, given at the dose of 500mg twice a day for at least 3 months. To ensure full absorption, both have to be taken at least

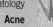

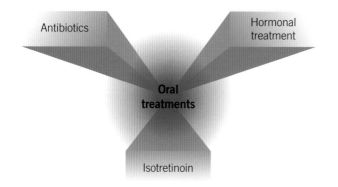

Fig. 7. The three main oral treatments for mild-to-moderate acne.

40 minutes before food with a glass of water. A Cochrane review[2] found that while minocycline is effective for moderate acne, there was no reliable evidence to justify its use as a first-line treatment, given its price and concerns about side-effects (pigmentation and, rarely, a lupus-like syndrome).

If there has been no improvement after 3 months, erythromycin can be tried at the same dosage for the same length of time. It may be the first choice of treatment for women who may become pregnant or who are breastfeeding. Trimethoprim is another possible choice.

Using different topical and systemic antibiotics at the same time encourages resistant strains of *P. acnes*.

Hormonal treatment

Co-cyprindiol (cyproterone acetate with ethinylestradiol) is no more effective than an oral antibiotic, but may be worth considering for women with hirsutism as well as acne or who need an oral contraceptive. It contains an anti-androgen and so should be avoided during pregnancy.

Isotretinoin

This is a toxic drug that can only be prescribed by hospital dermatologists. Its main action is to reduce sebum production, sometimes by as much as 90%. It is used mainly for severe acne, but should also be considered if the acne:

- Has improved by less than 50% after 6 months of conventional oral antibiotic therapy.
- Relapses quickly after other treatment.
- Is mild but still causes scarring.
- Is mild but causes psychological distress.

Isotretinoin has many side-effects (Figure 8), and these should be discussed with the patient before treatment starts. The two most important are teratogenicity and depression.

> ❝ *Co-cyprindiol contains an anti-androgen and so should be avoided during pregnancy* ❞

> ❝ *Isotretinoin has many side-effects. The two most important are teratogenicity and depression* ❞

13

Fig. 8. Other side-effects of isotretinoin.

Side-effect	Proportion of patients affected
Chapped lips	95%
Dry skin and itching	80%
Dry nose/nose bleeds	80%
Irritation of the eyes	40%
Joint and muscle pains	15%
Temporary hair thinning	10%
Diminished night vision	<1%
Depression and suicidal thoughts	<1%

Teratogenicity

Effective contraception should be used for 1 month before starting treatment and for at least 1 month after treatment stops. Pregnancy must be excluded by a test 2 to 3 days before expected menstruation. If negative, treatment can start on day 3 of the menstrual cycle. The drug should also be avoided during breastfeeding, and those taking it should not give blood for transfusion. Before starting treatment, it is wise to ask women to sign a form confirming that they are not pregnant and have been warned about the risks. In Europe, following an EU ruling, specialists presribing isotretinoin to females of childbearing age will be required to check for pregnancy on a monthly basis, and may only issue the drug for a maximum of thirty days at a time.

> *Depression and suicide: patients should be warned about this before treatment starts*

Depression and suicide[3]

Patients should be warned about this before treatment starts, and told to stop the treatment immediately if there is any concern on this score.

Dosage and monitoring

The starting dose is usually 0.5mg/kg body weight. If the response is good after 1 month, this dose will be continued for a further 2 to 3 months. If the response is not satisfactory, the dose can be raised to 1mg/kg, again given for a further 2 to 3 months.

Whether patients should be investigated regularly during treatment is debated.[4] Most agree that a full blood count, liver function tests and fasting lipid levels should be measured before treatment starts and after one month. Changes in liver enzymes or lipid profiles occasionally warrant stopping the treatment. Other clinicians perform the same tests again after 10 and 16 weeks, and one month after the course has finished.

Isotretinoin is not guaranteed to cure acne permanently, although it has revolutionized acne treatment and many patients remain clear after taking it. Approximate relapse rates are shown in Figure 9.

Future developments

Possibilities include the use of long-term but low-dose isotretinoin regimens, and new anti-inflammatory agents such as lipo-oxygenase inhibitors. If more laboratories could check the antibiotic sensitivity of acne organisms, treatment could be tailored better to individual patients.

66 Isotretinoin is not guaranteed to cure acne permanently, although it has revolutionized acne treatment 99

Fig. 9. Approximate relapse rates after taking isotretinoin.

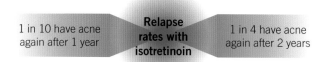

1 in 10 have acne again after 1 year

Relapse rates with isotretinoin

1 in 4 have acne again after 2 years

ACTINIC KERATOSIS

Introduction

Actinic, or solar, keratoses are common signs of ageing and environmental damage to the skin. They are capable of transformation into a squamous cell carcinoma (see page 98), although the potential for this in any one lesion is low. On the other hand, skin cancers of all kinds are more common in individuals with large numbers of actinic keratoses.

66 Actinic, or solar, keratoses are common signs of ageing and environmental damage to the skin 99

Definition and epidemiology[1]

An actinic keratosis is an area of dysplastic epithelium, but the histological changes do not amount to malignancy. Each patch is discrete, but the areas wax and wane suggesting that there is a "field change" varying from time to time between being relatively normal at one end of the spectrum to significant dysplasia at the other.

Actinic keratoses occur predominantly on sun-exposed skin and increase in frequency with age. Those with high lifetime levels of sun exposure (outdoor workers, avid sunbathers) have more than those with lower exposure and develop them earlier. Fair-skinned people are particularly at risk. Men with thinning or absent hair often have many actinic keratoses on their scalps.

Aetiology

Although ageing increases the tendency for skin cells to become dysplastic, the main factor is sun exposure. Immunosuppression (especially post-transplant) is becoming increasingly important.

15

Fig. 10. Treatment choices for actinic keratoses.

Treatment of actinic keratoses	
Small numbers	Liquid nitrogen cryotherapy
Large numbers or the frequent eruption of new lesions	5-fluorouracil Diclofenac Retinoic acid Imiquimod Photodynamic therapy
Large, fixed lesion	Curettage and cautery
Diagnostic uncertainty	Biopsy/excise

Diagnosis

Typically, actinic keratoses are scaly patches, often on a red background. Some become elevated and hyperkeratotic. One distinct variant is a slightly scaly, spreading pigmented patch.

As described above, lesions wax and wane, but there may be little change and there comes a point when the possibility of something more significant, such as a squamous cell carcinoma, should be considered. Deciding this on clinical grounds alone may be almost impossible and histology is usually required. However, even under the microscope, the distinction between a highly dysplastic actinic keratosis and a well-differentiated squamous cell carcinoma can be difficult to make. In practical terms, diagnosis and treatment are achieved by this approach and the outcome will be the best possible.

The distinction between a pigmented actinic keratosis and a lentigo maligna (see page 66) is more clear-cut histologically.

❝ The distinction between a pigmented actinic keratosis and a lentigo maligna is more clear-cut histologically ❞

Treatment

The choice of treatment for an actinic keratosis depends on several factors (see Figures 10 and 11).

The choice may vary from the box options, depending on individual patient factors, including preference.

❝ Avoiding sun exposure limits further damage. Patients should watch out for persistent skin lesions, which may be skin cancers ❞

Prevention

Avoiding sun exposure limits further damage. Patients should watch out for persistent skin lesions, which may be skin cancers. Actinic keratoses predispose specifically to the development of squamous cell carcinomas, but basal cell carcinomas and melanomas (especially lentigo maligna melanoma) are also more frequent in skin showing multiple lesions.

Use of treatments for actinic keratoses	
Liquid nitrogen	A relatively gentle freeze will deal with most lesions.
5-fluorouracil[2]	The cream should applied daily for up to 3 weeks and then the applications should be stopped. There is often a brisk reaction and patients may need to suspend treatment earlier. Inflammation can be controlled with topical steroids if necessary. Care must be taken to avoid contact with eyes. Alternative regimens have been proposed, using 5- fluorouracil alternately with topical steroids, or on an intermittent basis, such as for 2–3 days each week.
Retinoic acid	Daily application may control and reduce visible actinic keratoses. It is rather an irritant.
Diclofenac	Daily application (up to 4 weeks) may control and reduce visible actinic keratoses.
Imiquimod	Daily application (6–8 weeks) may control and reduce visible actinic keratoses.
Photodynamic therapy	Only available in selected centres currently. UV radiation following application of a photoactivated chemical destroys the actinic keratoses. It can be painful.
Curettage	It is simple to curette and cauterize an actinic keratosis under local anaesthetic.
Biopsy/excision	Either part or the whole of the lesion is removed under local anaesthetic and submitted for histology.

Fig. 11. How to use the various treatments for actinic keratoses.

ALOPECIA AREATA[1]

Introduction

There are many causes of hair loss. One of the most striking, and easiest to diagnose, is alopecia areata and its more extensive variants alopecia totalis and alopecia universalis.

Definition and epidemiology

The term *alopecia areata* is reserved for the common condition in which circumscribed patches of hair loss appear, often quite suddenly, over areas of apparently normal skin. If the changes extend to the whole scalp, the term *alopecia totalis* is employed, while *alopecia universalis* is reserved for the rare event in which all scalp and body hair is lost.

Aetiology

"Aetiology: the changes are thought to be induced by an autoimmune attack on the hair follicles"

The changes are thought to be induced by an autoimmune attack on the hair follicles (and/or the pigment within the hairs), and this may be, at least in part, genetically determined. There is often a family history of the condition, or of vitiligo, or both. Patients and their relatives are also more likely to have organ-specific autoantibodies (for example to thyroid, adrenal or gastric parietal cells), and there may be a family history of diabetes, thyroid disease and pernicious anaemia. This is not true of all patients, however.

The disorder affects adults and children. Some have lesions, on and off, throughout their lives, and the most unfortunate may lose some or all of their hair permanently.

Diagnosis

A typical case is unmistakable. One or more patches of hair loss appear, usually on the scalp, but quite often affecting the eyebrows and eyelashes: indeed the loss of eyebrow or eyelash hair is virtually pathognomonic of alopecia areata. The patches spread, often quite rapidly, before arresting, stabilizing and, in most cases, beginning to regrow. Regrowing hair is often white initially, and may never repigment. At the edge of an active lesion it is usually possible to find short, tapered hairs known as "exclamation mark hairs" (Figure 12). These are absolutely diagnostic.

"The more severe forms of the condition can lead to permanent and extensive hair loss"

The skin of the scalp is generally completely normal on inspection, although patients frequently complain of some tingling or itching. Occasionally the scalp is a little reddened and care has to be taken to exclude a fungal infection in a child.

As indicated above, the more severe forms of the condition can lead to permanent and extensive hair loss.

Prevention

"There is no known way of preventing the progress of this disorder"

There is no known way of preventing the progress of this disorder.

Treatment[2]

Topical steroids are often used initially, but whether they make much difference is a moot point. Intradermal injections of triamcinolone

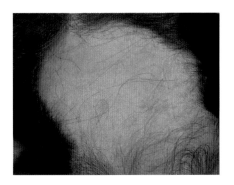

Fig. 12. Alopecia areata. Exclamation mark hairs can be seen at the right edge of this area. Reproduced with kind permission from Graham-Brown R and Bourke JF. Mosby's Colour Atlas and Text of Dermatology. London: Mosby Ltd, 1999.

directly into patches do seem to aid recovery, but are logistically only possible with relatively limited disease. Over-use, and/or subcutaneous injection may lead to atrophy. A burst of systemic steroids is occasionally justified for extensive, rapidly progressive changes but, although this may arrest and reverse the process for a while, the disease usually progresses again once the steroids are stopped.

One other alternative is available, and involves the deliberate induction of a contact dermatitis on the affected areas, usually with diphencyprone. This is normally carried out only in a specialist unit. If all else fails, patients will need advice and help obtaining appropriate hairpieces or wigs.

ARTEFACTUAL SKIN DISEASES

Introduction

These skin lesions are caused by patients themselves, sometimes with the intention of deceiving others. They range from the results of common habits, such as nail biting, to the skin lesions of those whose delusions make them believe they are harbouring parasites. Figure 13 describes the more common forms. Figure 14 shows a chemical burn that was caused intentionally by a patient.

❝Artefactual skin lesions are caused by patients themselves, sometimes with the intention of deceiving others❞

Condition	Comments
Habit tic nail dystrophy	Common. An unconscious habit of rubbing the cuticles leads to a ladder pattern of transverse ridges and furrows running up the centre of a thumbnail.
Nail biting	Common. Short nails with a ragged free edge. Hard to treat. Minor degrees are common, mainly in middle-aged women.
Neurotic excoriations	Lesions are scabbed, usually less than 1cm across and seen, mixed with scars, on the face, neck and back. Antidepressants help some patients.
Lip licking	Crusted, bleeding lips resulting from persistent biting and licking.
Hair pulling habit	Trichotillomania is too strong a word for what is usually a transient habit seen in children under stress. Sometimes the wisest course of action is to ignore it.
Excoriated acne	Seen mainly in females, and stress related. The lesions are pick marks that leave scars, and may be based on trivial acne lesions. Isotretinoin treatment is occasionally justified.
Delusions of parasitosis	Rare. Patients are convinced that they are infested. This is usually just a "single hypochondriacal delusion", but they cannot be persuaded otherwise. They move from doctor to doctor, complaining of incompetence. The "parasites" turn out to be non-specific fragments. Skin lesions are dig marks. It is best not to agree with the patient about their delusion, but to try to persuade them to take pimozide if it is not contraindicated by ECG abnormalities.
Dermatitis artefacta	The intention here is to deceive. The secondary gain may be attention, time off work or money. Lesions appear suddenly, in easily accessible areas, and do not look much like any recognized skin disorder. Some take up odd shapes, such as those left by drips of corrosive fluid running down the skin.
Dermatological pathomimicry	This is the deliberate aggravation of a skin disorder, for example by the self-application of an allergen to which patients know they will react.
Habituation to dressings	Elderly men who like attending for dressings on their legs, even though their ulcers healed long ago.

Fig. 13. A synopsis of artefactual skin disorders.

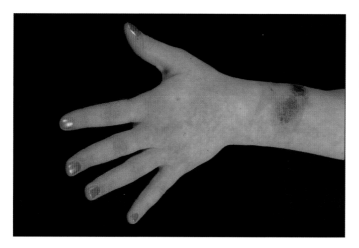

Fig. 14. Chemical burns on the forearm of a teenage girl who was suffering problems at school.

BASAL CELL CARCINOMA

Introduction

Basal cell carcinomas are the commonest skin cancers and, although UK registration data are poor, are also the most common malignant tumour in white-skinned people. Fortunately, basal cell carcinomas rarely metastasize, although local invasion can be troublesome, especially around sites such as the eyes, ears and nose.

❝ Basal cell carcinomas are the commonest skin cancers ❞

Definition and epidemiology

A basal cell carcinoma is a malignant proliferation of epidermal keratinocytes, with a very low metastatic potential, but capable of direct invasion and destruction of adjacent tissues (Figure 15).

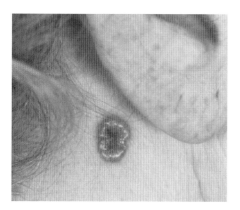

Fig. 15. A typical basal cell carcinoma below the ear.

21

Variants of basal cell carcinoma	
Solid/nodular	Lesions begin as small translucent papules. As they expand, a central depression frequently develops and leads to an annular appearance. Telangiectatic vessels over the surface are a highly characteristic feature.
Cystic	Cystic lesions are prominent with marked translucency.
Morphoeic	The greater stromal, connective tissue element is reflected in a flat or depressed area, looking like a scar.
Superficial	Especially common on the trunk. Lesions are indolent, reddish areas with a fine, serpiginous edge, often flecked with pigment. They continue to expand for years, leaving irregular, roughened skin centrally, but occasionally larger nodular elements may arise .
Pigmented	Occasionally basal cell carcinomas are heavily pigmented.

Fig. 16. Clinical variants
of basal cell carcinoma.

Aetiology

Like the other skin cancers, basal cell carcinomas are more common in the elderly, and are also linked to sun exposure. The quantity of UV in childhood may be particularly important.

Diagnosis

A number of clinical variants are recognized (see Figure 16). A good pointer to the diagnosis is contact bleeding (probably due to superficial telangiectases), and any facial lesion showing this should be considered suspicious. Most tumours occur on the head and neck, although the superficial variant favours the trunk, and lesions on the limbs are not as rare as once they were.

The definitive diagnostic test is histology.

Avoiding excessive sun exposure should reduce the incidence of basal cell carcinomas over time

Prevention

Avoiding excessive sun exposure should reduce the incidence of basal cell carcinomas over time.

Treatment[1,2]

The best treatment for most basal cell carcinomas is adequate excision, although clearance can be difficult to assess in morphoeic lesions.

Some specialists advocate other measures, such as 5-fluorouracil, curettage and cryotherapy, especially for superficial basal cell carcinomas, but these are not appropriate for lesions in the high-risk locations around the eyes, nose and ears. Radiotherapy is effective but far more time-consuming than excision.

BOWEN'S DISEASE

Introduction

In situ squamous cell carcinoma occurs in the skin, as it does in cervical and other epithelia. For historical reasons this change on non-genital skin is referred to as "Bowen's disease". *In situ* squamous cell carcinoma of the female genitalia is managed by gynaecologists. Dermatologists, however, do become involved in the management of the same changes on the penis, where the *erythroplasia of Queyrat* is a form of Bowen's disease.

Definition and epidemiology[1]

Bowen's disease is squamous cell carcinoma *in situ*. It is seen mainly in older patients, on sun-exposed sites.

> *Bowen's disease is squamous cell carcinoma in situ*

Aetiology

The most common cause is UV radiation, although patches may develop over time in anyone. Lesions also occur:

- In those who have been treated in the past with arsenic.
- On areas of skin exposed to other ionizing radiation, especially X-rays.
- In association with human papilloma virus infections.

Other known aetiological agents include immunosuppression, especially after transplantation.

> *The most common cause is UV radiation*

Diagnosis

At first sight, a patch of Bowen's disease looks rather like psoriasis (Figure 17). However, the surface scale is thicker and less flaky, and there is no bleeding when this scale is lifted off. Instead there is a moist, red surface. The diagnosis may need a biopsy. Similar changes occur on the penis, almost exclusively in the uncircumcised.

> *At first sight, a patch of Bowen's disease looks rather like psoriasis*

Prevention

Avoiding precipitating factors is important. Invasive squamous cell carcinoma can develop at any time in a patch of Bowen's disease, although this is uncommon in clinical practice. However, substantial changes in an area of Bowen's disease must be biopsied.

Fig. 17. Patch of Bowen's disease. Note the close resemblance to psoriasis. Reproduced with kind permission from Graham-Brown R and Bourke JF. Mosby's Colour Atlas and Text of Dermatology. London: Mosby Ltd, 1999.

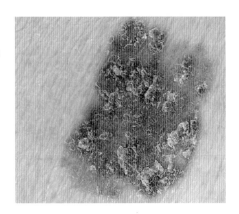

Treatment[2]

The range of therapies is similar to that used for actinic keratoses (see page 16), although small single patches of Bowen's disease are excised more often than keratoses. Bowen's disease is common on the lower leg, where cryotherapy may lead to poor healing.

CANDIDIASIS

Introduction

66 The yeast Candida albicans is present in the mouths of about 40% of the population 99

The yeast *Candida albicans* is present in the mouths of about 40% of the population, and in the vagina of 10% of women. It is not carried on normal skin but, as an opportunistic pathogen, easily takes advantage of the changes listed under "Aetiology" to establish itself there.

The lesions caused by candida vary with the site of infection (Figure 18).

Aetiology

Candidal infections of the skin are more likely in the presence of:

- Diabetes, obesity, poor hygiene, high humidity (predispose to candidal intertrigo).
- Pregnancy, oral contraceptives, conjugal spread (predispose to genital candidiasis).
- Prolonged immersion of the hands in water by people with poor peripheral circulation (predispose to candidal paronychia, finger web candidiasis).
- Medications such as antibiotics and corticosteroids (all types of candidiasis).
- HIV infection.

Site	Appearance of candidiasis
Occluded major flexures (candidal intertrigo)	Moist, glazed erythema, with soggy scaling at the edge, and outlying "satellite" papulopustules.
Genital candidiasis	An itchy vulvovaginitis, with white plaques adherent to inflamed mucous membranes. After conjugal spread, similar lesions can appear under the foreskin.
Oral candidiasis	Adherent white plaques on the mucous membranes. Red sore areas under dentures.
Paronychia	Chronic rather than acute. Lost cuticles, bolstered red nail folds exuding small amounts of pus if squeezed, adjacent nail becomes ridged and discoloured.

Fig. 18. The commonest types of mucocutaneous candidiasis.

Systemic candidiasis (seen in patients with immunosuppression or leucopoenia) and chronic mucocutaneous candidiasis (seen in inherited defects of immunity, hypoparathyroidism, Addison's disease, a low serum iron, and thymic tumours) are both rare and outside the scope of this book.

Diagnosis
Swabs from the affected area should be sent for culture. Urine should be tested for sugar.

66 Urine should be tested for sugar 99

Treatment[1]
Treatments for cutaneous candidiasis are described in Figure 19.

DERMATOFIBROMA

Introduction
Another common benign tumour of human skin is the dermatofibroma (also known as histiocytoma). These are generally no more than a nuisance but must be differentiated from a cutaneous malignancy.

66 Dermatofibroma must be differentiated from a cutaneous malignancy 99

25

Treatment	Indication	Measures to be used
Measures to alter local susceptibility factors	Cutaneous and oral candidiasis	• Oral – denture hygiene, leave dentures out at night. • Skin flexures – careful drying and powdering, skin fold separation. • Hands – keep warm and out of water.
Local anti-candidal therapy	Will suffice for most cutaneous candidiasis without internal predisposing factors	• Skin – a topical imidazole antifungal preparation (clotrimazole, econazole, ketoconazole, miconazole, sulconazole) or nystatin. Combinations with a mild corticosteroid help candidal intertrigo. • Mouth – infants: nystatin suspension or miconazole gel applied several times a day. Others – oral nystatin pastilles or suspension, amphotericin lozenges, or miconazole oral gel.
Oral treatment	For refractory cases	• Oral itraconazole or fluconazole. Both are convenient quick ways of treating vaginal candidiasis.

Fig. 19. Treatments for cutaneous candidiasis.

Definition and epidemiology

A dermatofibroma is a collection of spontaneous scar tissue, with the elements of the scar varying in amount from lesion to lesion. The histopathology is characteristic.

Dermatofibromas are extremely common, particularly in women, and have a predilection for the legs, although they can occur anywhere. It is not uncommon for several lesions to appear on different sites and at different times.

Aetiology

Many seem to follow minor skin trauma, such as an insect bite or a thorn prick. However, there may be no preceding history.

Diagnosis

Typical lesions are easy to diagnose clinically. They are small, firm dermal nodules, usually round with a smooth surface. They move

66 *Typical lesions are small, firm dermal nodules, usually round with a smooth surface* 99

within the skin and are wider than they are deep, being lozenge-shaped in cross-section. Their overall shape and size is not unlike that of a lentil. Lesions may itch or hurt on contact, presumably because of nerve entrapment within the tumour.

Their colour ranges from pale pink to quite dark (the pigment being haemosiderin, not melanin), and dark ones can give rise to diagnostic difficulty. They should be removed for histology if there is any doubt.

Treatment
Many need no treatment. If they are symptomatic, unsightly, or if there is diagnostic doubt, they should be excised.

66 Dermato-fibromas many need no treatment 99

DERMATOPHYTE INFECTIONS

Introduction
The treatment of dermatophyte infections was revolutionized in the late 1950s by griseofulvin, and more recently by terbinafine and the imidazole antifungals. Despite this, some types are on the increase. Up to 20-fold increases in scalp ringworm, for example, have been recorded in large cities in the UK.[1] The subject remains important.

Definition and epidemiology
Dermatophyte fungi invade the keratin of the stratum corneum, the nails and hair. The clinical picture depends on the site of the infection, the type of fungus, and the inflammatory response (see Figure 20).

66 Dermatophyte fungi invade the keratin of the stratum corneum, the nails and hair 99

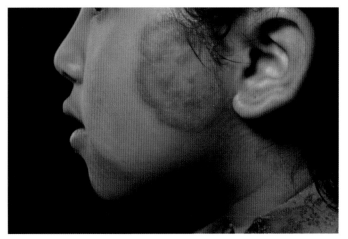

Fig. 20. A friendly hamster passed on this ringworm infection.

27

> *66 Tinea pedis affects up to 70% of the adult population worldwide 99*

Estimates vary, but all agree that dermatophyte infections are common. At least 15% of the UK population have tinea pedis, which affects up to 70% of the adult population worldwide. The prevalence of scalp ringworm is rising both in the US and in the UK, where a recent study of London schoolchildren showed a prevalence of 2.5%, and carriage rates of up to 47%.[1]

Aetiology

Dermatophytes can be subdivided in several ways:

- Into those that live on animals as well as humans (zoophilic), and those that infect humans only (anthropophilic). In general, the former stimulate a greater inflammatory response than the latter. An

Fig. 21. The diagnosis and management of scalp ringworm.[2]

Clinical type	Diagnosis	Management
• Until recently most UK cases were due to *Microsporum canis* (from infected dogs or cats). • Currently *T. tonsurans* (spread from child to child) tops the list in most cities. • In the country, a kerion (due to *T. verrucosum* from cattle, highly inflamed and capable of leaving a scarred bald area) should be considered. • Favus (due to *T. schoenleinii* and characterized by yellow cupped crusts) is rare in the UK.	• The diagnosis is easy to miss as the mixture of signs is so variable (patchy alopecia, broken hairs, scalp scaling, pustules). Consider it in any child with a scaly scalp thought to be an unresponsive dandruff or scalp eczema. • Wood's light reveals a green fluorescence only in microsporum infections. • Always send scalp scrapings and broken hairs to a mycology laboratory.	• The source of the infection must be dealt with. A vet can treat an infected pet. In anthropophilic infections, classmates should be examined and specimens sent to the laboratory. • Tinea capitis requires systemic treatment, but in the UK griseofulvin is the only drug licensed for this purpose in children, although terbinafine and itraconazole are effective. • An antifungal cream should be used as well as systemic therapy. • A child on adequate oral and topical therapy is safe to return to school.

Clinical type	Diagnosis	Management
There are three main clinical patterns of tinea pedis: 1. Soggy scaling in lateral toe webs. 2. Recurrent episodes of vesication. 3. Dry diffuse scaling of soles and sides of feet ("moccasin foot"). This may be associated with similar changes on one palm. Usually due to *T. rubrum*.	• Made by examining scrapings microscopically and sending them for culture. • The differential diagnosis of toe web maceration includes erythrasma, bacterial overgrowth, and soft corns. • Suspect a chronic *T. rubrum* infection, and examine the feet, if a patient complains of having one dry scaly palm.	A topical imidazole or terbinafine preparation usually suffices. However, for the dry *T. rubrum* type, oral treatment (for example with terbinafine or itraconazole) is also needed. Terbinafine works faster than griseofulvin but costs more. Itraconazole and fluconazole work just as well.[3]

Fig. 22. The diagnosis and management of tinea pedis.

extreme example is a kerion (a scalp infection with cattle ring-worm), which is so inflamed that it looks like a carbuncle.

- Into three genera : trichophyton (skin, hair and nail infections), microsporum (skin and hair) and epidermophyton (skin and nails).

Diagnosis and management

Each type of dermatophyte infection has a characteristic appearance, and needs different management.

Topical therapy may be all that is needed for mild fungal infections. Most cases of tinea cruris and tinea corporis, for example, will respond to it. If not, systemic therapy is needed.

Suggestions for managing fungal infections in particular areas are given in the Figures 21, 22 and 23.

66 Each type of dermatophyte infection has a characteristic appearance, and needs different management 99

Clinical type	Diagnosis	Management
There are three patterns: 1. Yellow crumbliness and thickening starting at the free edge and working proximally. This is the commonest type. 2. The "superficial white" type, with white powdery patches on the surface away from the free edge. 3. Proximal subungual type, seen especially in patients with AIDS. This is a generally white but minimally thickened nail.	• Consider psoriasis, paronychia, and onycholysis. • Clippings should be sent to the laboratory for microscopy and culture.	• Topical applications of amorolfine lacquer or tioconazole solution succeed only in mild limited onychomycosis. • Usually systemic treatment is needed, but do not start this without laboratory confirmation of the diagnosis. • Terbinafine (the first choice of treatment: for adults 250mg daily for 6 to 12 weeks) and itraconazole (pulsed therapy with 400mg daily for 1 week of each month for 2 months for fingernails and 3 months for toe nails) both have higher cure rates than griseofulvin and may help with non-dermatophyte fungi that can invade damaged nail plates. • Unlike griseofulvin, terbinafine and itraconazole are not licensed for use in nail infections of children.

Fig. 23. The diagnosis and management of tinea of the nails.[4]

DISCOID LUPUS ERYTHEMATOSUS

Introduction

Although classified as lupus erythematosus, the problems of discoid lupus erythematosus do not stem from the involvement of internal organs. They come from the ugliness of the skin lesions, which are most common on the face (Figure 24), and from scars and pigmentary changes left behind if treatment is delayed or ineffective.

Definition and epidemiology

Discoid lupus erythematosus and systemic lupus erythematosus lie at opposite ends of the spectrum. One is localized to the skin, the other is a severe multisystem disorder. Subacute cutaneous lupus erythematosus is a subset lying between the two extremes. Discoid lupus erythematosus seldom changes into systemic, and most sufferers from it are otherwise healthy.

Discoid lupus erythematosus is:
- Twice as common in women as in men.
- Chronic, although about half of patients go into remission after several years.

Its prevalence in the population is not known accurately.

Aetiology

Discoid lupus erythematosus is considered an autoimmune disease: the incidence is higher in those with certain HLA combinations. It is exacerbated and sometimes triggered by ultraviolet light.

❝ Discoid lupus erythematosus and systemic lupus erythematosus lie at opposite ends of the spectrum. One is localized to the skin, the other is a severe multisystem disorder ❞

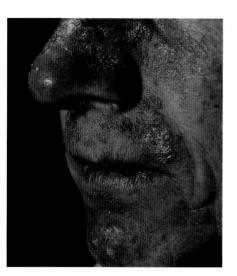

Fig. 24. Discoid lupus erythematosus. Classical lesions on the face. The red scaly areas show marked follicu lar plugging. Reproduced with kind permission from Savin JA, Junter JA and Hepburn N. Diagnosis in Color: Skin Signs in Clinical Medicine. London: Mosby Ltd, 1997.

31

Diagnosis

The diagnosis can be made by recognizing a mixture of the following physical signs in well-demarcated plaques on exposed areas:

- Erythema and telangiectasia
- Scaling
- Follicular plugging
- Pigmentary changes (most marked in coloured skin) include hypopigmentation centrally and hyperpigmentation peripherally
- Scarring and loss of hair, most marked in scalp lesions

❝ It is wise to confirm the diagnosis by a biopsy ❞

It is wise to confirm the diagnosis by a biopsy. Direct immunofluorescence shows deposits of IgG, IgM, IgA, and C3 at the basement membrane. Screening blood tests for systemic lupus erythematosus are also worthwhile.

The differential diagnosis includes psoriasis (this can be confused with subacute cutaneous lupus erythematosus), "Jessner's lymphocytic infiltration of the skin" (turgid erythematous plaques that lack scaling and follicular plugging, and which may be a dermal form of discoid lupus erythematosus), and polymorphic light eruption (see page 77).

Treatment

A Cochrane review[1] drew three rather cautious conclusions from 54 studies of the treatment of discoid lupus erythematosus:

1. *"High potency fluorinated steroid creams may be superior to low potency hydrocortisone."* Clinical experience supports this strongly.

2. *"Both hydroxychloroquine and acitretin are associated with marked improvement or clearing in about half of all people treated, although neither drug has been tested against placebo. Adverse effects such as dry lips were troublesome in nearly all people in the acitretin group."* Hydroxychloroquine is now preferred to chloroquine as it carries less risk of ocular side-effects, which are rare anyway on current low-dose regimens.

❝ Most clinicians also advise patients to avoid the sun and to use a sunscreen regularly ❞

3. *"At present there is no reliable evidence to support the use of other specific treatments for discoid lupus erythematosus. This should not be seen as evidence that current treatment is ineffective but rather that evidence of effectiveness is lacking."*

Most clinicians also advise patients to avoid the sun and to use a sunscreen regularly.

ECZEMA/DERMATITIS

Atopic eczema

Introduction

Atopic eczema is a common inflammatory condition affecting all age groups, but it usually presents in childhood (Figure 25).

Definition and epidemiology

Complicated lists of features have been devised to define atopic eczema for research purposes, but the key clinical features that most experts would accept are listed in Figure 26. Most patients will have all of these.

There are no diagnostic laboratory tests, although sufferers often have high levels of circulating IgE, and positive skin prick tests to common allergens.

Atopic eczema is common and, in western societies, becoming more so in recent years. Population-based studies indicate that 20% or

66 Sufferers often have high levels of circulating IgE, and positive skin prick tests to common allergens 99

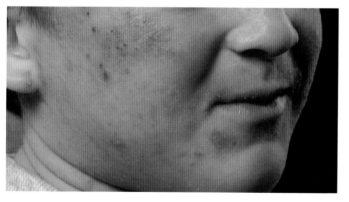

Fig. 25. Typical atopic eczema showing the important complication of widespread *H. simplex* infection.

Fig. 26. Features of atopic eczema.

Definition of atopic eczema
Patients will have or have had:
• Itch
• The actual presence or a history of flexural eczema (the face can be considered a "flexure" in babies)
• A personal or family history of eczema, asthma or hay fever

33

more of children in the UK now develop at least mild atopic eczema before age 4.[1] No particular ethnic group is favoured, but the disease is most common in those at the higher end of the social ladder.

About 60–70% of patients clear before adolescence, but recurrences are not uncommon later in life. It is impossible to predict who will clear, or at what age. However, in general, the more severe the eczema and the stronger the family history of persistence, the worse the prognosis.

Aetiology

" Atopic eczema has a strong genetic basis "

Atopic eczema has a strong genetic basis[1]: the high rate of affected family members indicates this, and twin studies confirm it. There are numerous abnormalities, including alterations in the way the immune system responds to external stimuli and differences in epidermal lipids. However, it is not clear whether genetic predisposition alone dictates when or whether the disease appears. Environmental triggers play an important role and there is much speculation as to what these are, and how they operate.

The environment could affect atopic eczema in a number of ways.

Early-life exposure

An early-life exposure could initiate a cascade of changes that become self-perpetuating. Popular candidates include substances in the infant's or mother's diet.

Absence of early-life exposure

" Some clinicians speculate that a low exposure to "dirt" and infection in infancy explains the rising prevalence "

The absence of early-life exposure could also allow abnormalities to develop. Some clinicians speculate that a low exposure to "dirt" and infection in infancy explains the rising prevalence of atopic eczema (the "hygiene hypothesis").

Repeated exposure

Repeated exposure to environmental factors could prolong or exacerbate the disease. There are many potential candidates here, including diet, aeroallergens such as pollens, and house dust mites.

" The jury remains "out" on the cause of the skin changes in atopic eczema "

None of these theories, however, is fully supported by current evidence and the jury remains "out" on the cause of the skin changes in atopic eczema. This has not prevented a wide range of doctors from engaging in therapeutic interventions based on their interpretation of what might be important, and many parents, carers and patients are very keen to identify what is "causing" the disease.

Diagnosis

As indicated above, there are some key features that most, if not all, patients will have. There are also a number of other helpful clinical signs.

- In babies the face is prominently involved, with red, inflamed skin. Similar changes appear over the trunk and limbs, often on the extensor surfaces.
- In older children there is an increasing tendency for flexural surfaces to become involved (antecubital and popliteal fossae, wrists and ankles).
- The skin becomes thickened and rough ("lichenified") especially over the wrists, hands, ankles and feet.
- A similar phenomenon occurs around the eyes, where the "Dennie–Morgan" infraorbital fold is commonly seen.
- Patients with atopic eczema often have a generally dry skin. The term "xerosis" is often used for this, but many have changes amounting to ichthyosis.
- There may be multiple scratches and abrasions. Patients have feverish bouts of scratching; some children seem never to stop rubbing and scratching at their skin.
- Weepy, yellow, impetiginized crusts are commonly caused by infection with *Staphylococcus aureus*.

> **" Patients with atopic eczema often have a generally dry skin "**

Eczema herpeticum

Superinfection with the herpes simplex virus can be devastating in patients with atopic eczema. Viral lesions spread widely over the skin surface, creating an appearance like chicken pox (hence the old name of "Kaposi's varicelliform eruption") (see Figure 25).

In a first attack there is a high swinging fever, and the patient is very unwell. This can be life threatening as explained in Figure 27.

> **" Superinfection with the herpes simplex virus can be life threatening "**

Prevention

There are many strongly held beliefs that altering diet, reducing exposure to various contact allergens or breastfeeding can prevent atopic eczema. However, the evidence is sketchy. More recently, a theory has been proposed that early stimulation of the immune system can reverse the changes that are seen in atopic eczema. Studies are being conducted with probiotics and various vaccines.

Treatment[2]

There is no switch-off cure, but realistic goals include moderation of the major symptom (itch) and an improvement in the major signs.

The main therapies employed in atopic eczema are listed in Figure 28.

> **" There is no switch-off cure "**

Fig. 27. How superinfection with herpes simplex virus can be life threatening.

Herpes simplex virus superinfection

The skin ceases to be an effective barrier; fluid and protein are lost, and metabolic disturbances follow

The skin becomes susceptible to invasion by bacteria that can cause septicaemia

Viraemia and viral encephalitis may occur

« The standard first-line treatment for atopic eczema is emollients »

The standard first-line treatment for atopic eczema is emollients applied to most or all of the body surface, except for the scalp. The choice of agent is highly individual: children, parents and physicians have their favourites. In theory, the heavier and greasier the emollient the better, but practical aspects dictate otherwise. Most families also use bath oils, although the evidence that they have much effect is limited. "Wet-wrapping", where the creams are applied under damp bandages, enhances the effect of emollients on a very dry skin, or on particularly active eczema in babies.

Inflammatory changes need more than emollients to achieve control. The best understood agents for this purpose are the topical corticosteroids. Unfortunately, fear among parents, nurses, doctors and the media has limited their acceptability for many. The oft-repeated adage "use the minimum amount of the weakest possible steroid" should in fact read: "use the minimum *effective* amount of the weakest possible steroids". It is often better (and may be safer) to use corticosteroids of a higher strength in short bursts, and to follow this with weaker ones, or even emollients alone for maintenance therapy. The new non-steroidal calcineurin antagonists, tacrolimus and pimecrolimus, may offer a useful alternative to steroids in mild eczema, or act as an "in-between" stage after emollients but before topical steroids, or vice versa. However, it is too early to be sure what role, if any, they will play.

« Use the minimum effective amount of the weakest possible steroids »

Secondary infection is common, although defining this is difficult because atopic eczema is often colonized by *S. aureus*. It is thought that the organism plays a pathogenetic role in some patients. Certainly,

Fig. 28. First- and
second-line treatment
for atopic eczema.

Treatments for atopic eczema	
First-line treatment	
Emollients	Liberal use keeps the skin comfortable and can reduce need for other modalities. Often used at bath time.
Corticosteroids	Highly effective but frighten many parents, nurses and doctors. Often best used in bursts, when higher potency agents may establish control and weaker ones can then be used for "maintenance".
Anti-infectives	Useful if there is suspected secondary infection.
Tar	Very soothing and very safe. This treatment is underused. Available in cream or bandage formulations.
Antihistamines	Non-sedating ones are of little benefit. Sedating ones assist sleeping and reduce nocturnal scratching.
Calcineurin antagonists (tacrolimus, pimecrolimus)	Very new. May assist in reducing amount of topical steroid needed. Good for face and flexures.
Second-line treatment (best initiated/monitored by a specialist)	
Photo- and photochemotherapy	Can be very helpful. Some skin cancer risk.
Immunosuppressive drugs	Ciclosporin is highly effective. Reserved for very severe disease.
Environmental manipulation	Attempts to change diets are common but usually haphazard and potentially harmful. Reduction of house dust mites may help but requires enormous effort.

judicious use of a short course of antibiotics can often improve the skin significantly, but the longer-term use of oral or topical anti-infective agents is controversial and not backed by good evidence.

When atopic eczema cannot be helped adequately by such simple measures, the "second-line" approaches listed in Figure 28 should be considered. They are usually best initiated by a specialist.

"Judicious use of a short course of antibiotics can often improve the skin significantly"

37

Special mention must be given to environmental manipulation, especially changes in diet and avoiding house dust mites, because both are thought to be useful by many "authorities" in contact with patients and their families. As a consequence, dietary manipulation is extremely common and, despite advice from all experts, is frequently started without input from a dietician. This is potentially hazardous. Furthermore, the evidence that diet affects atopic eczema is limited, although it is true that reactions to foods, such as contact urticaria, are common. The same is true of contact with animal fur, grasses and some pollens. Randomized trials suggest that reducing levels of house dust mites may improve atopic eczema.

❝ Reducing levels of house dust mites may improve atopic eczema ❞

Eczema herpeticum needs active treatment with an intravenous antiviral agent in a first or severe infection, but oral therapy may be satisfactory for recurrent attacks.

Contact dermatitis[1]

Introduction
Eczematous skin changes may be due, wholly or partly, to direct contact with external factors. This is contact dermatitis.

Definition and epidemiology
Contact dermatitis is the induction or exacerbation of eczematous skin lesions as a result of direct contact with an external agent or agents. There are two recognized forms (Figure 29).

Fig. 29. The two forms of contact dermatitis.

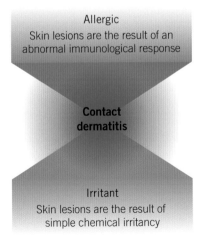

Allergic
Skin lesions are the result of an abnormal immunological response

Contact dermatitis

Irritant
Skin lesions are the result of simple chemical irritancy

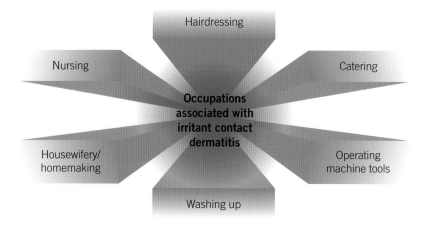

Fig. 30. Occupations and activities commonly associated with irritant contact dermatitis.

Aetiology
Primary irritant dermatitis
The skin can withstand a degree of chemical insult but, if exposure is prolonged, the materials are particularly harsh, or the individual is especially sensitive, an irritant dermatitis may develop. This occurs most easily in those with an "endogenous" eczematous tendency, such as atopic eczema. Common irritants include soaps, detergents, shampoos (especially in hairdressers), foodstuffs and cutting oils. Simply working with constantly wet hands may induce the same changes.

Occupations notorious for their high prevalence of irritant contact dermatitis are shown in Figure 30.

It often takes repeated injury over time for the reaction to develop but, once started, short breaks from exposure only give short-lived remissions followed by rapid deterioration.

❝ Common irritants include soaps, detergents, shampoos (especially in hairdressers), foodstuffs and cutting oils ❞

Contact allergic dermatitis
Some people develop a type IV, delayed, cell-mediated hypersensitivity to allergens. Thereafter, exposure even to minute quantities of the offending agent induces dermatitis predominantly at the site of contact. These reactions begin within the epidermis when antigens, present on the surface of the Langerhans cells, trigger a T-cell response.

Many agents can induce contact allergic dermatitis. Some are listed in Figure 31.

Antigen	Common pattern/site(s)	Environmental source
Nickel and cobalt	Eczema under jewellery, watches and fastenings	Non-precious metals
Chromates	Hands and/or feet, face (due to airborne contact)	Cement, tanned leather, industrial processes
Rubber chemicals	Hands, forearms, waist, feet	Gloves, shoes, elasticated materials
Colophony	Under sticking plasters	Sticking plasters
Phenylenediamines	Face, especially eyelids, which are often oedematous	Hair dyes
Formaldehyde, the "parabens" group, ethylenediamine, quaternium 15	Almost anywhere but often eyelids and face. May complicate varicose eczema and otitis externa	Preservatives in medicaments and toiletries
Lanolin	Anywhere. May complicate varicose eczema and otitis externa	Medicaments and toiletries
Aminoglycosides (especially neomycin)	Anywhere. May complicate varicose eczema and otitis externa	Medicaments
Corticosteroids	Anywhere	Medicaments
Plant antigens	Linear streaks at point of contact, face (due to airborne contact)	Primula obconica (UK), Rhus (poison ivy) (USA), Parthenium (India), Chrysanthemum spp and many others
Wood antigens	Hands, forearms, face (due to airborne contact)	Hardwoods, especially mahogany

Fig. 31. Agents that cause contact allergic dermatitis.

Diagnosis

Investigation must start with a careful history of exposure to potential sensitizers. It is important to establish any possible work or domestic sources, including details of tasks carried out, hobbies and leisure pursuits, and of cosmetics, toiletries and medicaments being applied to the skin. It is also often useful to test to materials suspected by the patient (for example make-ups and materials handled at work). However, care must be taken not to place highly irritant chemicals on the skin.

It may also be worth visiting the place of work. Often this draws attention to tasks and contacts not apparent from the history alone.

66 Investigation must start with a careful history of exposure to potential sensitizers 99

Primary irritant dermatitis

The possibility that irritant factors are playing a role in initiating or exacerbating eczema should always be considered, and a history of occupational and domestic exposure should be a fundamental part of the initial consultation.

Contact allergic dermatitis

Contact allergy should be suspected in a patient with dermatitis at the sites mentioned in Figure 31. However, "secondary" spread to adjacent, or even to distant non-contact sites, is common and may cause confusion. Certain sites are more often secondarily affected than others. This is especially the case for eyelids, which are commonly inflamed in metal sensitivity.

Volatile material, or material that can be blown around as dust, can cause "air-borne" contact dermatitis. This involves the face, backs of hands and other exposed areas, simulating a light-sensitive eczema (see page 76). However, the classic light-spared areas are usually affected.

The key investigative technique is patch testing. Suspected offending agents are applied to the surface of the skin for 48 hours, and the site is examined for evidence of allergic dermatitis. A second reading at 72 or 96 hours is also worthwhile as some compounds produce late reactions. In most instances, a battery of common test allergens is used and this can be modified for local circumstances and for particular problem areas or occupations.

66 The key investigative technique is patch testing 99

66 Avoiding irritants and exposure to potential sensitizers is good practice 99

Prevention

Avoiding irritants and exposure to potential sensitizers is good practice for anyone with a history of eczema or "sensitive" skin.

Treatment[2]

66 *The only permanent solution to contact dermatitis is to stop exposure to the provoking material* **99**

The only permanent solution to contact dermatitis is to stop exposure to the provoking material or activity, but this is not always possible. Relief can also be obtained by judicious use of topical corticosteroids to suppress inflammation, liberal use of emollients and non-soap cleansers, and protecting the skin with gloves and barrier creams.

Discoid eczema

Introduction

66 *Patients of all ages may present with round or oval patches of eczema* **99**

Patients of all ages may present with round or oval patches of eczema, unrelated to any other recognized diagnostic category. An alternative name is "nummular" eczema (from the Latin for a small coin).

Definition and epidemiology

The term "discoid eczema" is used for round or oval patches of eczema with no other identifiable cause. It is common, especially in elderly men. A high alcohol intake may be a risk factor.

Aetiology

No clear-cut cause has been identified.

Diagnosis

Typical patches are not a problem (Figure 32), but they can be confused with psoriasis and fungal infections, although these days discoid eczema is a more common cause of inflamed red rings than tinea.

Fig. 32. Widespread, itchy, erythematous lesions in a 55-year-old woman.

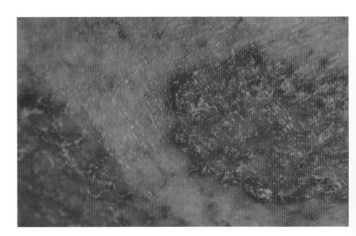

A biopsy will confirm eczema if there is any doubt, and it may sometimes be prudent to send a sample for mycology.

Treatment

Topical corticosteroids are the mainstay of therapy, but new lesions usually continue to erupt at random, even if there is a good initial response. If these are tackled early, they can usually be eradicated rapidly. If not, UVB phototherapy can be helpful. Secondary bacterial infection is common and the combined use of steroids with antiseptics or even antibiotics may be more effective than steroids alone.

“Topical corticosteroids are the mainstay of therapy”

Seborrhoeic eczema

Introduction

The term seborrhoeic eczema is applied to two different conditions:
1 A common disorder of adults that presents with redness and scaling in a typical distribution (see Figure 33).
2 A less common condition seen in infants, known as "infantile seborrhoeic dermatitis". Here, severe cradle cap accompanies dermatitic changes in the flexures and napkin area.

Definition and epidemiology

Seborrhoeic eczema is common, affecting both sexes. The adult form is not seen before puberty and is particularly common in patients with HIV infection.

“Particularly common in patients with HIV”

Aetiology

There is good evidence that a commensal yeast (Pityrosporum) plays a role in provoking the skin lesions in some patients.

Sites of predilection of seborrhoeic eczema
• Scalp
• Eyebrows
• Nasolabial folds
• Retroauricular groove
• Mid-chest and back
• Axillae
• Infra-mammary folds
• Groins

Fig. 33. Typical distribution of seborrhoeic eczema in adults.

43

Diagnosis

The diagnosis is based on the typical clinical features (see Figure 34) and on the exclusion of key differential diagnoses, the most important being flexural psoriasis (see page 86).

Prevention

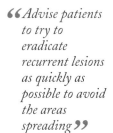

66 Advise patients to try to eradicate recurrent lesions as quickly as possible to avoid the areas spreading 99

Advise patients to try to eradicate recurrent lesions as quickly as possible to avoid the areas spreading.

Treatment[1,2]

A cream containing a mild-to-moderate corticosteroid and an azole (for example miconazole or clotrimazole) often controls the lesions, but they will recur. Preparations containing lithium succinate are also effective. Scalp lesions respond to topical corticosteroids, but strong ones are generally required. Adding salicylic acid also helps. Shampoos containing zinc pyrithione, selenium sulphide or ketoconazole are also useful.

In severe seborrhoeic eczema, a short course of oral itraconazole may be worth trying. Tacrolimus and pimecrolimus are reported to be useful and do not cause skin atrophy even after prolonged use.

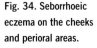

Fig. 34. Seborrhoeic eczema on the cheeks and perioral areas.
Reproduced with kind permission from Graham-Brown R and Bourke JF. Mosby's Colour Atlas and Text of Dermatology. London: Mosby Ltd, 1999.

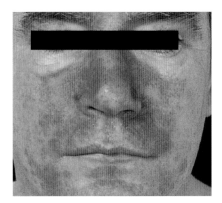

Varicose (stasis) eczema

Introduction

66 The condition is defined as eczema due to underlying venous disease 99

Patients with venous disease, with or without evident varicose veins, can develop eczematous changes on their lower legs, and occasionally elsewhere.

Definition and epidemiology

The condition is defined as eczema due to underlying venous disease. Its exact prevalence is unknown, but venous disease is common.

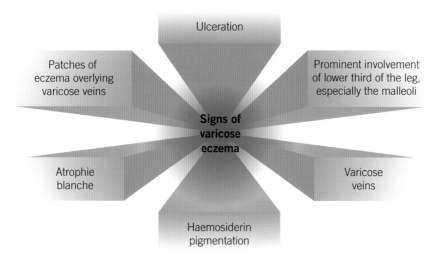

Fig. 35. Signs indicating a diagnosis of varicose eczema.

Aetiology

There is no doubt that eczematous changes can be due to venous disease, but the mechanisms involved are not understood.

Diagnosis

Any eczematous area on the lower leg should be viewed as possible varicose eczema. The diagnosis will be supported by the presence of any or all of the signs shown in Figure 35.

Venous insufficiency can be confirmed by duplex scanning of the leg veins. A positive result does not, of course, mean that the eczema is inevitably venous.

Occasionally, the changes become much more extensive, spreading over wide areas of the body. This suggests a secondary contact allergic dermatitis (see page 41), a major problem in a chronic condition for which so many treatments are used.

" Venous insufficiency can be confirmed by duplex scanning of the leg veins "

Treatment and prevention

Initial relief should be sought from topical corticosteroids. Potent ones may be needed for very active eczema. It is important to avoid potential contact sensitizers in the medications, notably antibiotics and antiseptics (especially aminoglycosides, clioquinol/chlorquinaldol), and base constituents, including lanolin, parabens and other preservatives.

It may be wise to avoid anything present in the patient's current treatment if possible.

If and when control is achieved, further investigation should include an assessment by a vascular surgeon, as surgery might be appropriate. Doppler studies will establish whether the arterial supply to the legs is adequate and capable of supporting compression (see "Leg ulcers", page 108). If a contact allergic dermatitis is suspected, the patient should be referred for patch testing (see "Contact dermatitis", page 38).

ERYSIPELAS

Introduction

« Erysipelas is potentially lethal »

Erysipelas is potentially lethal. It must be diagnosed and treated quickly with little help from the laboratory. Usually it does well, but recurrences are common and often a nuisance for years afterwards.

Definition and epidemiology[1]

« An attack is ushered in by bouts of shivering, malaise and high fever »

Erysipelas is an acute infection of the dermis and upper subcutaneous tissue, usually by beta-haemolytic streptococci of group A (Figure 36). An attack is ushered in by bouts of shivering, malaise and high fever. An erythematous area, with a well-defined margin, then appears and enlarges, accompanied by pain, and sometimes by lymphangitis or lymphadenopathy. Blisters, some haemorrhagic, can develop on the red area.

Fig. 36. A febrile patient with hot, spreading, haemorrhagic patches due to a streptococcal infection.

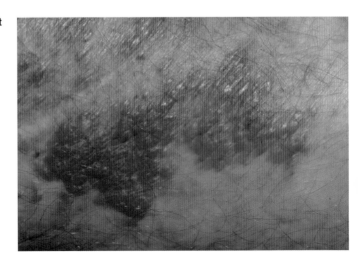

Factors predisposing to erysipelas	
Disruption of the epidermal barrier	• The commonest (about 60%) are toe web fissures, either from macerated intertrigo or tinea pedis • Leg ulcers, pressure sores, wounds • Leg dermatoses
General factors	• Lymphoedema • Venous insufficiency • Obesity • A knee prosthesis or a previous varicose vein operation • Factors of debatable relevance include alcoholism, diabetes and smoking
Factors favouring a longer than average hospital stay	• Development of blisters • Presence of leg ulcers • Old age
Predisposing to recurrence	• Persistence of toe web fissuring and maceration • Lymphoedema

Fig. 37. Some factors predisposing to erysipelas.

Before antibiotics were readily available, the commonest site was the face and the mortality rate was high. Now, 90% of lesions are on the legs and the death rate is less than 1%. About a fifth of patients have recurrences.

❝ 90% of lesions are on the legs ❞

Aetiology

Figure 37 lists some predisposing factors. The commonest is a fissure in a toe web, and the most important internal one is lymphoedema. About a quarter of patients with limb lymphoedema experience at least one episode of a skin infection such as erysipelas.[2] In contrast, the figure for the general population is about 1 in 1000.

Diagnosis

No diagnostic test is specific for erysipelas but, before starting treatment, it is worth sending blood for culture as well as surface samples from the inflamed area, particularly from blisters. However, the yield of positive results is relatively low.

Conditions to distinguish from erysipelas include:

- Cellulitis: this is a subcutaneous infection that has less sharp margins than erysipelas.
- Necrotizing fasciitis: this is an emergency needing a deep biopsy and surgical debridement. It starts as a dusky area like cellulitis. It is more painful, and there is disproportion between the shocked state of the patient and the lack of local signs.
- Venous thrombosis.

Treatment

Patients should have bed rest with the affected limb elevated. Many patients are treated in hospital, staying an average of 10 days. There is no advantage in using antibiotics other than penicillin (or erythromycin for penicillin-allergic patients). With penicillin, patients become apyrexial in 24 to 48 hours, and the local symptoms and signs settle over about a week.

For mild cases, a course of oral penicillin V suffices, with the addition of flucloxacillin if a staphylococcal infection is suspected. For more severe cases, intravenous benzylpenicillin can be used.

Long-term, low-dose penicillin V (250 to 500mg a day) cuts down the frequency of attacks in recurrent erysipelas. Anticoagulants can be given to patients at risk of a deep vein thrombosis. The risk of recurrence drops if the portal of entry is treated vigorously.

66 There is no advantage in using antibiotics other than penicillin 99

HEAD LICE

Introduction

Many parents are shocked when their children catch head lice, and the shock turns into despair if the infestation proves hard to clear. However, treatment will be successful if the right insecticide is picked, and enough attention is paid to detail.

66 Treatment will be successful if the right insecticide is picked 99

Definition and epidemiology

Head lice are parasitic insects adapted to living on the human scalp and neck hairs, which they grasp with their modified legs. They are host-specific. To survive, they have to feed on their host's blood several times a day.

The prevalence of head lice is not known precisely, but perhaps 10% of children in the UK carry them. Many have no symptoms and itching, the main symptom of infestation, can take 3 months or more to develop.

Characteristics of head lice are given in Figure 38.

Aetiology

Adult lice are greyish and roughly 3-4mm long. They spread from head to head by direct contact, and rarely via shared hats or combs. Their eggs stick firmly to the shafts of hairs. Some details of their life cycle are given in Figure 39.

"Spread from head to head by direct contact"

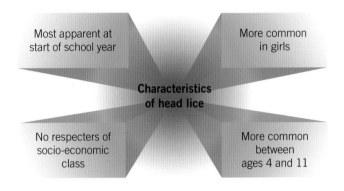

Most apparent at start of school year

More common in girls

Characteristics of head lice

No respecters of socio-economic class

More common between ages 4 and 11

Fig. 38. Typical characteristics of head lice.

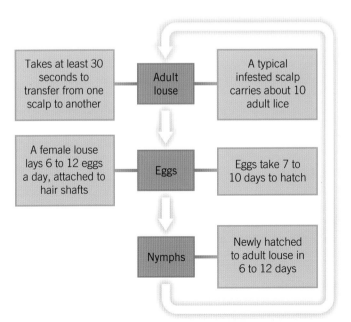

Takes at least 30 seconds to transfer from one scalp to another

Adult louse

A typical infested scalp carries about 10 adult lice

A female louse lays 6 to 12 eggs a day, attached to hair shafts

Eggs

Eggs take 7 to 10 days to hatch

Nymphs

Newly hatched to adult louse in 6 to 12 days

Fig. 39. The head louse and its life cycle.

Fig. 40. Conditions that may be confused with head lice infestation.

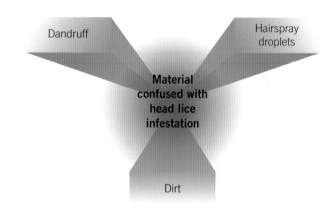

Diagnosis

The diagnosis should always be considered in recurrent scalp or face infections. Differential diagnoses are given in Figure 40.

"Imaginary lice" can accompany psychogenic itch.

The presence of living, moving lice is required to diagnose a current infestation needing treatment. Empty egg shells (nits) alone indicate a past infestation and need observation only. Louse droppings show up as black specks on collars or pillows.

" Empty egg shells (nits) alone indicate a past infestation and need observation only "

Prevention

The key points to note in preventing infestations are:

- It is not a good idea to use insecticides prophylactically. This encourages resistance.
- The value of louse repellents containing piperanol is uncertain.
- It may be worth combing the hair regularly to detect an early infestation.
- Curing infested patients is a waste of time unless close contacts are traced, and treated if infested.
- There is no need to exclude children with head lice from school.

" There is no need to exclude children with head lice from school "

Treatment

A Cochrane review[1] found that physical methods of cure (for example, combing or bug busting) are less effective than using a pediculicide. There was no evidence that one pediculicide is more effective than another. The best choice of treatment depends on knowing local resistance patterns.

" Physical methods of cure are less effective than using a pediculicide "

Pediculicides

The pediculicides of choice are malathion, the synthetic pyrethroids (phenothrin and permethrin) and carbaryl. Two applications should be used, 7 to 10 days apart, so that the second one kills lice hatching out after the first application. If live lice are found on follow-up, a pediculicide from another chemical class should be used. Occasionally a third choice may be needed.

Formulations include alcohol-based lotions (effective and less likely to produce resistance, but irritant and to be avoided in young children and those with eczema or asthma), and aqueous liquids. At least 50ml are needed for each application, and should be left on for at least 12 hours. Shampoos may be less effective.

> ❝ *Two applications should be used, 7 to 10 days apart* ❞

Other measures
Louse combs can be used to remove nits and dead lice after treatment. Combs, brushes, pillows, hats and so on should be cleaned.

Reasons for treatment failure are given in Figure 41.

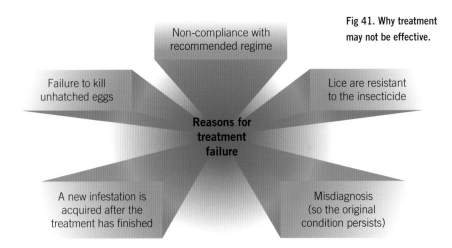

Fig 41. Why treatment may not be effective.

Non-compliance with recommended regime

Failure to kill unhatched eggs

Lice are resistant to the insecticide

Reasons for treatment failure

A new infestation is acquired after the treatment has finished

Misdiagnosis (so the original condition persists)

HERPES SIMPLEX

Introduction
At least 85% of the world population have serological evidence of having had a herpes simplex infection. Many pass the virus on even when they have no obvious active infection, by "asymptomatic viral shedding". The so-called "quiet pandemic" will be with us for a while.

> ❝ *At least 85% of the world population have had a herpes simplex infection* ❞

Definition and epidemiology
Herpes simplex infections can be primary – the first infection in a previously seronegative patient – or recurrent. The two are separated by a latent phase (Figure 42.)

51

Clinical stage	Features
Primary infection	• Follows direct contact with an infected individual, either with active disease or shedding viral particles during a latent phase. • An acute gingival stomatitis in children is the most common type. • Genital herpes simplex is also common. • Other manifestations include a "herpetic whitlow" on a fingertip, and innoculation herpes elsewhere. • Primary episodes are usually more severe than recurrences. • Complications include eczema herpeticum, dissemination in the immunosuppressed, and encephalitis.
Latent phase	• This is lifelong, despite treatment. • The virus persists in sensory nerve ganglia. • Virus particles may be shed asymptomatically.
Recurrent infections	• Virus is reactivated and travels peripherally in sensory nerve fibres. • Trigger factors include minor trauma, febrile illnesses, ultraviolet light, and possibly stress. • Replication in the skin or mucous membrane then creates a recurrence. • The commonest sites are the face and genitals. • Complications include: erythema multiforme (65% of attacks are triggered by a herpes simplex recurrence within the preceding 2 weeks), eczema herpeticum, persistent ulceration in the immunocompromised, and keratoconjunctivitis.

Fig. 42. The phases of herpes simplex infection.

Infections are least common in the highest socio-economic classes. By age 30, 50% of adults of high socio-economic status in the US are seropositive to HSV-1, in contrast to 80% of those of lower status.

Aetiology

Two types of herpes simplex virus are recognized: HSV-1 and HSV-2. They are closely related but differ in their epidemiology, although both are spread by close personal contact.

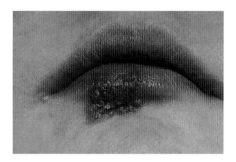

Fig. 43. Typical coldsore due to an *H. simplex* infection. Reproduced with kind permission from Graham-Brown R and Bourke JF. Mosby's Colour Atlas and Text of Dermatology. London: Mosby Ltd, 1999.

HSV-1 infections

These are usually acquired in childhood after contact with infected saliva (Figure 43). Most facial lesions are caused by HSV-1.

Features typical of recurrent HSV-1 infection are:
- A prodromal itch or tingling lasting a few hours.
- Groups of blisters that appear on an erythematous background.
- Infectivity is maximal for the first 2 days of an outbreak.
- Lesions arise in the same general area, but not in exactly the same place each time.
- Scabbing follows vesication. Healing takes 5 to 7 days, and usually leaves no scar or permanent loss of sensation.

❝HSV-1 infections are usually acquired after contact with infected saliva❞

HSV-2 infections

These are transmitted sexually, and begin to appear at puberty, or are spread from a mother's genital tract infection to a newborn child. Most genital infections are caused by HSV-2.

Some features are:
- The longer a primary infection lasts, the more frequent are the recurrences.
- The median recurrence rate is about one attack every 3 months for HSV-2 infections (and far less often for genital HSV-1 infections). Recurrence rates decrease with time.
- Recurrences are harmful psychologically.

❝HSV-2 is transmitted sexually❞

Prevention

Prevention is difficult because the virus is ubiquitous and spread by people with no obvious active infection. Also, about 80% of genital herpes is transmitted when there is no sign of infection. Regular use of condoms helps prevent genital herpes and a high protection factor sunscreen helps to prevent recurrent facial lesions.

Those looking after patients with atopic eczema should stay away if they have cold sores because eczema herpeticum is so serious.

Suppressive long-term antiviral therapy may be needed for particularly frequent or severe relapses.

❝Those looking after patients with atopic eczema should stay away because eczema herpeticum is so serious❞

Treatment

Mild outbreaks do not need treatment. The introduction of aciclovir (an inhibitor of herpes DNA polymerase) in the late 1970s was a milestone, although it does not eradicate the virus. The prevalence of aciclovir resistance in herpes simplex virus isolates from immunocompetent hosts has remained stable and low at 0.3%. The comparable figure for isolates from the immunocompromised is higher at 4-7%.[1]

Topical aciclovir and penciclovir creams shorten attacks if they are used early enough. Valaciclovir, a prodrug of aciclovir, and famciclovir, a prodrug of penciclovir, are as effective as aciclovir and need to be taken less often.

The decision to use oral antiviral therapy for recurrent facial herpes simplex depends on the frequency and severity of relapses, and the damage being done to the quality of life.

Long-term suppressive therapy can be considered in genital herpes relapsing more than 5 times per year. Vaccine therapy is still being evaluated.

ICHTHYOSIS

Introduction

The word "ichthyosis" comes from the Greek for fish. It refers to an abnormally dry and scaly state of the skin. In normal skin, surface keratinocytes are shed in such a way that the skin does not seem scaly, but in ichthyosis this does not happen (Figure 44).

❝Abnormally dry and scaly state of the skin❞

Definitions and epidemiology

The commonest type (ichthyosis vulgaris) affects about 1 in 300 of the population. A less common type, inherited as an X-linked recessive trait, is found in about 1 in 6000. Both persist throughout life. Less common still, and outside the scope of this book, are the ichthyosiform erythrodermas (mixtures of dryness and erythema).[1] Finally, an acquired type of ichthyosis has a variety of causes.

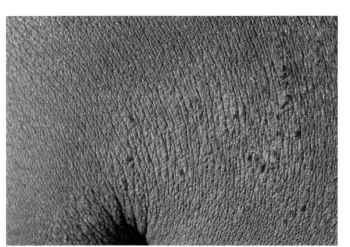

Fig. 44. An Afro-Caribbean child with a generally dry skin and a tendency to mild atopic eczema.

Aetiology

X-linked ichthyosis is due to a deficiency of steroid sulphatase. It affects males only. The responsible gene lies at Xp22.3, and in 1987 was the first to be identified in an inherited skin disorder.

Ichthyosis vulgaris is inherited as an autosomal dominant trait. The gene for one subtype may lie in the epidermal differentiation complex on chromosome 1.[2]

If ichthyosis appears in adult life (an acquired ichthyosis), the underlying cause is probably a lymphoma, usually Hodgkin's disease. Less often, malabsorption, chronic hepatic or renal disease, or an HIV infection underlie it.

“X-linked ichthyosis affects males only ”

Diagnosis

Figure 45 lists features that differentiate the two main types of ichthyosis.

Treatment

Treatment may not be needed in the summer when ichthyosis improves spontaneously. Otherwise consider:

- Maintaining a high humidity at home.
- Regularly applying emollients,[3] which soothe and smooth. The most severely affected prefer greasy preparations such as white soft paraffin, emulsifying ointment, or liquid and white soft paraffin ointment. They work best if applied after a bath or shower.
- Using bath oils and aqueous cream as a soap substitute.

“In the summer ichthyosis improves spontaneously ”

	Ichthyosis vulgaris	X-linked ichthyosis
Onset	Over first few months or years	Soon after birth
Scales	Small and branny, flexures spared	Larger and browner, flexures may be affected
Other features	• Accentuated skin creases of the palm • Keratosis pilaris is common	• Patients are often born after a prolonged labour • Corneal opacities in adult life • Testicular maldescent may occur

Fig. 45. Characteristics of the two most common types of ichthyosis.

IMPETIGO

Introduction

« The streptococcal type can sometimes trigger acute glomerulo-nephritis »

The word "impetigo" comes from the Latin for "an attack". Usually it attacks children, in whom the streptococcal type can sometimes trigger acute glomerulonephritis. This is its main danger.

Definition and epidemiology

Impetigo is not one condition, but a group of superficial contagious bacterial skin infections sharing several features (see Figure 46).

In the UK, GPs each year see about 3% of all children aged 0 to 4 and 1.5% of those aged 5 to 15 with impetigo.[1] This makes it the third most common skin condition in children (after eczema and warts). In developing countries the incidence is much higher. Outbreaks spread quickly through school classes and families.

Aetiology

Impetigo can be divided into its subtypes using the questions posed in Figure 46.

Diagnosis

« Always look for an underlying skin condition »

The diagnosis is made on clinical grounds (see Figure 47). Always look for an underlying skin condition, for example a scalp louse infestation provoking recurrent impetigo of the face and neck. A swab should be cultured for bacterial pathogens but treatment need not be delayed until the result comes back, particularly if you suspect a nephritogenic strain of streptococcus.

Questions	Answers
Primary or secondary impetigo?	• In primary impetigo, the bacteria invade normal skin. • In secondary impetigo, another skin disorder has disrupted the skin barrier, allowing impetigo organisms to establish themselves. Examples include impetiginized eczema, scabies, herpes simplex, and scalp louse infestations.
Bullous or non-bullous impetigo?	• The bullous type has larger blisters that rupture less readily, fewer lesions, and the trunk is often affected. • In the non-bullous type, the thin-walled vesicles rupture early to leave erosions covered in yellow or brown crusts. Mainly affects the face and limbs.
Staphylococcal or streptococcal?	• Bullous impetigo is always due to staphylococci. • Non-bullous impetigo is usually due to staphylococci, sometimes to a mixture of staphylococci and streptococci, and less often to streptococci alone. • Streptococcal impetigo is most common in hot humid conditions.

Fig. 46. Clues to the different types of impetigo.

Fig. 47. Annular patch of impetigo due to staphylococcal infection.

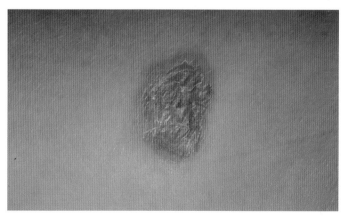

Prevention

In developing countries, encouraging the household to use an antiseptic soap reduces the incidence of impetigo.[2]

Treatment

The natural history of untreated impetigo has not been documented properly, and the best line of treatment has not been established.[3] Not surprisingly, opinions differ sharply. A middle of the road view is:

- For mild cases, removing crusts and exudate with an antiseptic such as povidone-iodine, plus regularly applying a topical antibiotic, may be all that is needed. Topical fusidic acid and mupirocin are popular as they are unlikely to be used systemically, and less likely than older topical antibiotics, such as neomycin, to cause allergy.
- For more widespread impetigo, a systemic antibiotic (usually flucloxacillin or erythromycin) should be used as well. Phenoxymethyl penicillin should be added to the flucloxacillin if you suspect a streptococcal infection.

KERATOACANTHOMA

Introduction

❝ Kerato-acanthomas are defined by their history of rapid growth and complete spontaneous resolution ❞

Keratoacanthomas are a pathophysiological curiosity. They are defined by their history of rapid growth and complete spontaneous resolution.

Definition and epidemiology

It is only possible to diagnose a keratoacanthoma definitively by waiting for it to disappear, although the histology of a typical specimen is characteristic (see below). Once it has been removed, of course, it is not possible to document the spontaneous disappearance on which the definition should rely.

Aetiology

❝ They usually appear on sun-exposed areas ❞

It is not known what triggers most keratoacanthomas, although they usually appear on sun-exposed areas, and may follow exposure to carcinogens such as tars.

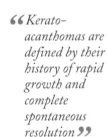

Fig. 48. A typical keratoacanthoma with a well-formed keratin plug.

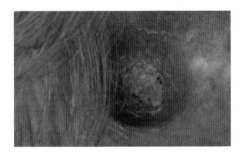

Diagnosis

The history of a rapidly growing lump, with a central, keratotic plug (Figure 48), is characteristic but not pathognomonic. It may be reasonable to await spontaneous resolution if the clinical signs are absolutely classical, but removal has the advantage of providing both diagnostic information and a cure.

"Removal has the advantage of providing both diagnostic information and a cure"

Prevention

Avoiding precipitating factors is prudent.

Treatment

The best approach is to remove the lesion by excision or curettage, although it may be reasonable to wait for 4 weeks or so, especially if the patient is very elderly or frail.

LICHEN PLANUS[1]

Introduction

Lichen planus is not particularly common, but is seen in general practice from time to time. Typical cases can be recognized immediately, but some variants are more difficult. The disorder is an autoimmune process, involving an interaction between the immune system and the skin.

"An autoimmune process, involving an interaction between the immune system and the skin"

Definition and epidemiology

While the clinical features of a classic case are unmistakable, most experts recommend histology as the best defining feature. There are no satisfactory estimates of the frequency of lichen planus in the general population, but it represents about 1% of new referrals to dermatology clinics. The figure quoted is, however, 4 decades old.

Aetiology

The underlying pathophysiology is clear. Lymphocytes attack the basal layer of the epidermis, leading to an unpredictable balance between destruction and repair. Shifts in this balance are reflected in the variability of the skin and mucous membrane lesions. Rarely, lichen planus is associated with other autoimmune diseases, but usually there is no underlying immunological disturbance.

It is not known what initiates the changes that lead to the skin lesions, but an environmental trigger may be responsible. The fact that lichen planus can be triggered and exacerbated by certain drugs supports this idea. However, a trigger cannot usually be identified.

"A trigger cannot usually be identified"

Common drugs that cause lichen planus-like rashes include:
- Beta blockers
- Antimalarials
- Thiazides
- Gold
- Penicillamine
- Phenothaizines
- Non-steroidal anti-inflammatory drugs

Diagnosis

In lichen planus, papules are scattered over the skin surface, with some sites of predilection (Figure 49). The condition may be extremely itchy, but is often surprisingly asymptomatic. Oral lesions may not be noticed until looked for at examination.

« The average time from onset to spontaneous disappearance is around 9 months »

The average time from onset to spontaneous disappearance is around 9 months, but some patients have more persistent disease or repeated attacks over many years. This is particularly true if the mucous membranes, or the hair and nails, are involved.

The features of classic lichen planus are listed in Figure 50.

Skin lesions

Cutaneous variants are listed in Figure 51.

Mucous membrane lesions

With mucous membrane lesions, the commonest change is a lacy network on the buccal surfaces. Gingivitis and atrophic or ulcerative changes may be seen, especially on the tongue. Chronic oral lichen planus predisposes to squamous cell carcinoma. Penile, vaginal, anal and oesophageal involvement also occurs.

Fig. 49. Extensive lichen planus in a classic site showing the violaceous colour. Reproduced with kind permission from Savin JA, Junter JA and Hepburn N. Diagnosis in Color: Skin Signs in Clinical Medicine. London: Mosby Ltd, 1997.

Hair and nails

Perifollicular lesions are difficult to diagnose (the term lichen planopilaris is applied to this condition). In the scalp, follicular lichen planus may result in a scarring (cicatricial) alopecia.

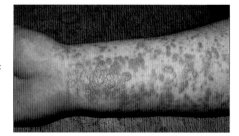

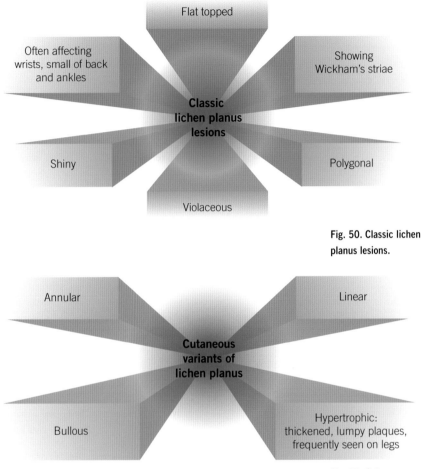

Fig. 50. Classic lichen planus lesions.

Fig. 51. Cutaneous variants of lichen planus.

Many patients have linear streaks in their nails. Severe involvement can lead to complete loss of nails.

Post-inflammatory hyperpigmentation
Lichen planus is noted for its tendency to leave pigmentary anomalies in its wake. This is particularly true in already pigmented skins.

Prevention
Patients with chronic oral disease should be kept under surveillance for the development of oral cancer.

Treatment[2]

Skin lesions respond, albeit slowly, to topical steroids

Skin lesions respond, albeit slowly, to topical steroids, but potent or very potent ones are needed to achieve much improvement.

Oral lesions are much more difficult to manage. There are various ways of delivering topical steroids to the oral mucosa (lozenges, special pastes, sprays), but the response is often indifferent and secondary candida infection is common.

Systemic therapy has a role when the lesions are spreading rapidly and very itchy, or when mucosal, hair or nail involvement is severe and threatens permanent damage. Oral prednisolone (or its equivalent) will usually arrest the disease but all too often the effect is temporary. Oral ciclosporin is an alternative.

LICHEN SIMPLEX

Introduction

Lichen simplex is also known as localized neurodermatitis

Lichen simplex is also known as localized neurodermatitis. The terminology may be awkward and archaic but, as the name implies, the concept is simple enough. These are patches of lichenification that would disappear if they were not scratched regularly and remorselessly. There is no underlying skin disorder.

Definition and epidemiology

Lichenification is due to rubbing and scratching

Lichenification is due to rubbing and scratching. The skin becomes thickened and leathery with increased surface markings. Well-established lichenification is usually darker than the surrounding skin.

Secondary lichenification is based on an itchy skin disease such as atopic eczema. In lichen simplex, however, the fixed itchy patches of lichenification arise *de novo*, always on easily reached areas, and are initiated and kept going by scratching, which is most fierce at times of greatest stress.

Other features include:
- Usually there is only one plaque, occasionally there are several.
- Peak incidence is between ages 30 and 50.
- Women are affected more often than men.
- Psoriasiform lesions on the nape of the neck are common in women but rare in men.
- Other common sites are the anogenital area and the outer calf.
- Paroxysms of scratching are most frequent at night.

Aetiology

Patients with lichen simplex develop scratch responses to minor stimuli more readily than controls. The original trigger for lichen simplex may have been as trivial as an insect bite, later the condition is self-perpetuating.

The paroxysms of scratching give pleasure when they start but become sore. Nevertheless, a bout of scratching can reduce itching for a while, although at the same time damaging the skin and liberating more pruritogens. This is the basis of the scratch/itch cycle.

Diagnosis

This is made on clinical grounds. A biopsy is seldom required. The commonest mistake is to misdiagnose lichen simplex on the nape of the neck as psoriasis. Confusion can also arise with patches of hyperkeratotic eczema and lichen planus.

Treatment

Measures that may help lichen simplex are given in Figure 52. Lesions can clear with treatment but tend to recur, in the same place or elsewhere, if the source of stress persists.

> *A bout of scratching can reduce itching for a while, although at the same time damaging the skin and liberating more pruritogens. This is the basis of the scratch/itch cycle*

Treating lichen simplex

1. Take a detailed psychological history – this may suggest ways of reducing tension.

2. Explain carefully the need to break the habit of scratching.

3. If the site allows, try occlusive bandaging, left on for several days at a time. This stops patients damaging their skin and helps to break the scratch/itch cycle. It is most effective on the limbs, but sometimes scratching starts elsewhere during treatment.

4. Use topical corticosteroid creams. Sometimes only potent ones will ameliorate the symptoms, as will infiltrating small plaques with triamcinolone.

5. Consider using a sedative antihistamine at night: tranquillizers and psychiatric treatment often disappoint.

Fig. 52. Treatment measures for lichen simplex.

MELANOCYTIC NAEVI

Introduction

Everyone has "moles". In the young, "moles" are usually melanocytic naevi. In older people, there is confusion because patients often apply the term wrongly to seborrhoeic warts and other pigmented excrescences. The main importance of melanocytic naevi lies in their relationship to malignant melanoma (see page 66), from which they have to be differentiated. In addition they can act as precursors to invasive malignant tumours.

Definition and epidemiology

Melanocytic naevi are embryonically derived collections of melanocytes. About 1% of babies have one or more melanocytic naevi

Fig. 53. Clinical variants of melanocytic naevi.

Variants of melanocytic naevi	
Congenital	Present at birth. Vary from small to giant/bathing trunk variant. The risk of melanoma is increased in large naevi, in smaller lesions the risk is not known.
Acquired	The classic "mole" has three phases – junctional, compound and intradermal. Usually begin as small, flat, brown areas. May thicken and eventually lose colour before disappearing altogether in the 6th, 7th and 8th decades.
Atypical/dysplastic	Larger with irregular shape and pigmentation. May show distinctive histological features. Can be a marker for genetic predisposition to melanoma.
Cockarde naevus	A naevus with a distinct ring of pigmentation around the edge.
Halo naevus	Mole surrounded by area of vitiligo. They are common. Naevus may disappear.
Spitz naevus	Common in children. Characteristic reddish/brown colour. Can be alarming histology at first glance.
Blue naevus	Blue/black colour may mimic melanoma, but lesions have smooth outlines and edges.

at birth. The rest of us develop them later, usually starting in childhood. Children growing up in sunny countries have more melanocytic naevi than those in colder climes.

Aetiology

It is assumed that most melanocytic naevi are chance aberrations of development, but a few families clearly have a genetic tendency to having large numbers, some of which are atypical (see below). There is also a link with sun exposure in childhood.

Diagnosis

Most common melanocytic naevi are easily recognized. There are also a number of recognizable clinical variants (Figures 53 and 54).

The main diagnostic task is to establish a negative. In other words, to determine that the pigmented lesion in question is not a melanoma. In this regard, the regularity of shape and pigmentation of most melanocytic naevi is reassuring. The greatest difficulty is encountered with "atypical" naevi: those with odd pigmentary changes, Spitz naevi and blue naevi. In these situations, and whenever there is real diagnostic doubt, excision for histology is the best approach.

66 Whenever there is real diagnostic doubt, excision for histology is the best approach 99

Treatment

Removal is indicated if there is diagnostic doubt, or if a lesion is unsightly and its removal will improve the appearance. We are not fans of using Lasers for melanocytic naevi.

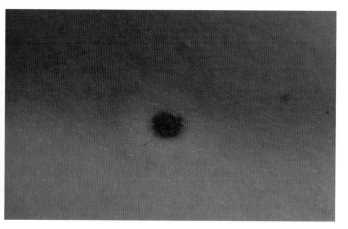

Fig. 54. Typical melanocytic naevus exhibiting the halo phenomenon.

MELANOMA (MALIGNANT)

Introduction

Malignant melanoma is cancer of melanocytes, which are the normal, pigment-producing cells. It is important because of its ability to metastasize, and because early recognition and removal can save lives.[1]

Definition and epidemiology

Malignant melanoma is not common in the UK when compared with breast or lung cancer, but its incidence has more than doubled over the past 3 decades.

Furthermore, although its incidence increases with age, malignant melanoma can and does affect young people, making it an important cause of mortality in those under 40. It is largely restricted to the white population: people of Asian or Afro-Caribbean descent are rarely affected.

Aetiology

66 Some families have a clear, genetic tendency to develop malignant melanoma with large numbers of abnormal naevi 99

The frequency with which malignant melanoma affects an individual (and a population) is closely linked to how much they are exposed to the sun, especially in childhood, and to the number of acute episodes of sunburn. Another risk factor is having large numbers of melanocytic naevi (see page 64), although this may also be partly due to high levels of childhood sun exposure.

Some families have a clear, genetic tendency to develop malignant melanoma. Most members of these families have large numbers of abnormal naevi (see page 64 and case study 2, page 121).

Diagnosis

Like all other cancers, a malignant melanoma develops from the expansion of a single errant cell. To recognize the diagnostic clinical features it is important to appeciate that this proliferation of malignant melanocytes can occur in a "radial" or a "vertical" growth pattern. Many start, and continue for some time, with a radial growth phase, spreading predominantly along the dermo-epidermal junction and upper dermis. Their vertical growth phase appears later. Others have no, or virtually no, radial phase and invade the dermis early.

This results in four distinct clinical subtypes of malignant melanoma.

Lentigo maligna (melanoma)

These are flat brown or black patches on sun-exposed skin. They occur especially in the elderly, but are increasingly seen in younger people. Lesions grow slowly over many years. The development of a nodule signals the fact that the lesion is beginning to invade the dermis.

Superficial spreading melanoma

This is the commonest form in the UK. At first the lesions are flat and grow slowly. They may occur anywhere, but are most common on the trunk in men and the legs in women. The development of a nodule suggests that the lesion has begun to invade the dermis (Figure 55).

Nodular melanoma

These are primary vertical growth phase tumours that may be difficult to diagnose accurately, although they usually present as relatively rapidly growing lumps.

Acral melanoma

These are rare, and the most prevalent type occurs in Asian and Afro-Caribbean patients. Lesions present as pigmented patches on the palms and soles, or as dark streaks in a finger or toenail, or nail fold, with or without destruction of the nail itself.

Diagnosis

Much has been written recently about diagnosing malignant melanoma. This has largely been in an attempt to help the public and non-specialist health professionals diagnose, or at least suspect, malignant melanoma more accurately. Figure 56 presents two "systems" that can help physicians and patients.

Certain signs are common in malignant melanoma. They relate to changes in size, shape and pigmentation, and to inflammation and symptoms. For the most part, changes in shape and pigmentation apply to the thin, radial growth phase forms of malignant melanoma,

66 Signs common in malignant melanoma relate to changes in size, shape and pigmentation, and to inflammation and symptoms 99

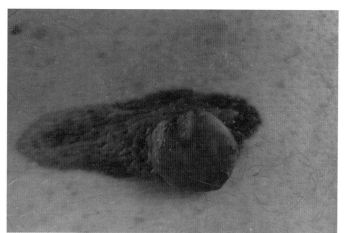

Fig. 55. If this superficial spreading melanoma had been removed earlier the invasive nodular component would not have developed.

Fig. 56. Two "systems" for diagnosing malignant melanoma.

Diagnosing malignant melanoma	
The ABCDE system*	**The seven-point check list^^**
Asymmetry	**Major**
	1. Change in size
Border (irregular)	2. Change in shape
	3. Change in colour
Colour variation	
	Minor
Diameter >6mm	4. Diameter >7mm
	5. Inflammation
Enlargement	6. Oozing/bleeding
	7. Itching
(*Esp. USA)	(**Esp. UK)

Fig. 57. The relationship between Breslow thickness and survival.

Breslow depth prognosis for malignant melanoma	
Breslow thickness	**Average 5-year survival**
<0.749mm	> 95%
0.75–1.49mm	>80%
1.5–3.49mm	60–70%
3.5mm	<40%

whereas inflammation, oozing and symptoms are more common in invasive vertical pattern tumours.

However, these features are not specific and or even diagnostic. Many benign skin tumours also trigger suspicion and still need to be examined by an educated pair of eyes, aided perhaps by magnification and refining techniques, such as "dermatoscopy".

Another key aspect of the diagnosis is its confirmation and assessment by histopathology. The pathologist should record the depth of invasion of the tumour using a specific measurement: the Breslow depth. This is the maximum depth of tumour cells from a fixed point in the epidermis. The prognosis of an excised malignant melanoma relates strongly to this figure (Figure 57). Such information can help a patient to understand the likely outcome.

Prevention

This relies on improved population education, early detection and early removal, although how successful these will be in the long-term is open to question. It is essential to follow-up high-risk families and individuals. Controlling sun exposure throughout life should reduce the number of tumours.

Treatment[2]

The only treatment that brings undoubted benefit is removal. It is perceived wisdom that incisional biopsies should not be performed on a suspected malignant melanoma and, because excision of suspicious lesions is generally straightforward, there seems no reason to disagree with this.

However, the same is not true of lentigo maligna when there is no clinical evidence of invasion, or of acral lesions, where making the diagnosis might lead to amputation, and accuracy is essential.

There are some areas of controversy:

- Wide excision: this is traditional, but there is little evidence that it improves survival. Most specialists offer advice and a degree of choice.
- Additional investigations: some specialists routinely perform further tests, such as a chest X-ray; others simply await the development of further signs of disease. There is an increasing trend towards radiological imaging and sampling of draining lymph nodes (sentinel node biopsy).
- Block dissection: random block dissection is no longer offered, but nodes may be removed after a sentinel node biopsy, or when there is obvious involvement.
- Radiotherapy, chemotherapy, and immunotherapy: most reserve these for recurrent disease, but some trials suggest a role for post-excision immunotherapy for some classes of tumour.

> *It is essential to follow-up high-risk families and individuals. Controlling sun exposure throughout life should reduce the number of tumours*

MOLLUSCUM CONTAGIOSUM

Introduction

In the nineteenth century many astute dermatologists, including Hebra, argued that molluscum contagiosum was not really contagious. They were wrong, of course, and today every doctor, school nurse and swimming pool attendant knows better.

Fig. 58. Cluster of molluscum contagiosum lesions in a typical site.

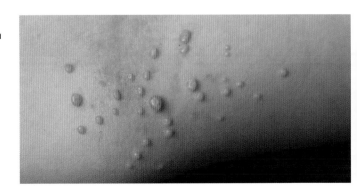

Definition and epidemiology

"Benign self-limiting condition " This is a benign self-limiting condition. Its firm, smooth, somewhat translucent papules can be skin-coloured, pink or pearly white (Figure 58). They have a central pore (umbilication) through which a cheesy plug can be squeezed out. Patchy eczema develops around the lesions of about 10% of patients.

Lesions range in diameter from 2mm to 6mm, and in number from 1 or 2 to a hundred or more. Usually there are fewer than 20. They can be grouped or widely disseminated. Numerous, stubborn and sometimes rather large lesions are seen in patients with sarcoidosis, lymphomas, leukaemia, atopic eczema and those on immunosuppressive therapy. The same applies to patients with HIV infection, 10% to 15% of whom have a molluscum contagiosum infection.

Molluscum contagiosum is most common in children under five (mainly on their trunk and limbs) and in sexually active young adults (often in areas that correlate with sexual contact, such as the lower abdomen, inner thighs, pubic area and genitals).

Mollusca can persist for months or years, but the average time for clearance is 6 to 12 months.

Aetiology

"Spread is through infectious debris during close personal, including sexual, contact " The causative organism is a large DNA pox virus, now separated into two subtypes (Figure 59).

Spread is through infectious debris during close personal, including sexual, contact. The incubation period is usually between 2 and 7 weeks, but can be longer. Other risk factors include swimming in a school pool and sharing a towel or sponge with an infected person.

Immunosuppression is important in determining the extent of the eruption. For example, in patients with an HIV infection, the severity of molluscum contagiosum is inversely related to the CD4 T-lymphocyte count.

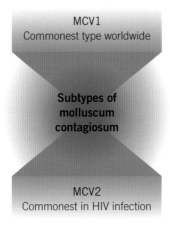

Fig. 59. The two subtypes of molluscum contagiosum.

Diagnosis

Mollusca are easily recognized. The differential diagnosis includes come-dones, milia, syringomas, and cellular naevi. Inflamed lesions can look like boils. Even senior dermatologists can mistake large single lesions for a keratoacanthoma or a basal cell carcinoma. Histologists enjoy com-menting on this. Surprisingly, mollusca are often confused with viral warts, which do not have a smooth surface or a central punctum.

In clinical doubt, material expressed from a punctum can be exam-ined, unstained, for typical large swollen epidermal cells, or stained to show up molluscum bodies. Alternatively, a whole lesion can be sent for routine histology.

Finally, it is worth checking patients with genital mollusca for other sexually transmitted disorders.

Prevention

It is not necessary to keep infected children away from school, but they should avoid swimming pools until they are clear. Skin-to-skin contact with infected individuals should be avoided, perhaps by using condoms and careful selection of sexual partners.

“ Infected children should avoid swimming pools ”

Treatment

Often treatment is not needed. Parents find this hard to believe, but the condition is self-limiting and many children learn their fear of doctors through attempts to squeeze out their multiple mollusca. It may be worth playing for time by suggesting a wart paint once a week to lesions well away from the eyes.

Most treatments are destructive. The easiest is to squeeze lesions with a pair of forceps, or to pierce them with an orange stick. Careful

“ Squeeze lesions with a pair of forceps, or pierce them with an orange stick ”

71

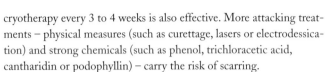

cryotherapy every 3 to 4 weeks is also effective. More attacking treatments – physical measures (such as curettage, lasers or electrodessication) and strong chemicals (such as phenol, trichloracetic acid, cantharidin or podophyllin) – carry the risk of scarring.

Recently, a topical immunomodulator (imiquimod cream) has been used with success, but is expensive and not for children. Systemic cidofovir can be considered for extreme cases, but has side-effects too and is expensive. Mollusca in patients with AIDS sometimes clear when highly active antiretroviral therapy (HAART) starts.

PAINFUL NODULE OF THE EAR

Introduction
Occasionally patients present with a small, tender nodule on the rim of one ear. The usual cause is an inflammatory condition, which has been given several names (for example, chondrodermatitis nodularis helicis), but which is best called a *painful nodule of the ear*.

Definition and epidemiology
"Almost exclusively in older patients"

Painful nodule of the ear is just that: a benign, tender swelling on the rim (helix), or occasionally the antihelix (Figure 60), of the pinna. It is more common in men than women and seen almost exclusively in older patients.

Aetiology
The condition is probably a pressure effect, leading to degeneration and inflammation in the cartilage and overlying skin.

Diagnosis
"Lesions are generally smooth and small, seldom more than 1cm"

Lesions are generally smooth and small, seldom more than 1cm in diameter, and often rather less. Patients complain of spontaneous discomfort or of pain on pressure, as when lying in bed on the side of the lesion. A gentle squeeze almost invariably reveals tenderness. The main differential diagnosis is a small basal cell or squamous carcinoma.

A typical example of painful nodule of the ear is unmistakeable, but if there is any doubt a biopsy or excision for histology is simple and diagnostic.

Treatment
Several approaches have their advocates, including excision, cryotherapy and intralesional injection with corticosteroids. Wedge excision under local anaesthetic is probably the most effective, but can cause minor

cosmetic deformity and so cryotherapy is often employed, at least at first. Intralesional steroid injections may be appropriate for the very frail.

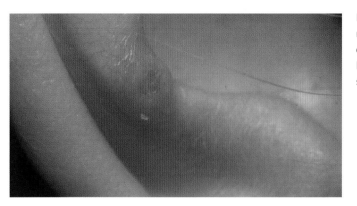

Fig. 60. A painful nodule on the antihelix of the ear. This is the less common of the two sites.

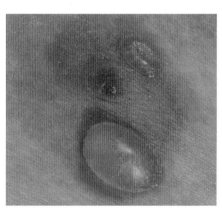

Fig. 61. A tense blister on an erythematous background. Reproduced with kind permission from Graham-Brown R and Bourke JF. Mosby's Colour Atlas and Text of Dermatology. London: Mosby Ltd, 1999.

PEMPHIGOID

Introduction

Pemphigoid is the commonest autoimmune blistering disorder. A quarter of those who have it die within a year, many from the side-effects of treatment.

Definition and epidemiology

Pemphigoid is a chronic blistering disease, mainly of the elderly. The average age at onset in one large series was 77. Blisters are subepidermal, usually arising on an urticarial background, and favouring the limb flexures and abdomen. Their roofs are formed by the whole thickness of the epidermis, so they can grow large and tense before rupturing (Figure 61).

" Pemphigoid is a chronic blistering disease, mainly of the elderly "

73

So unpleasant that active treatment is required

Although pemphigoid usually remits within a year or two, the symptoms are so unpleasant that active treatment is required. In the past this was usually with systemic corticosteroids.

Aetiology

Pemphigoid is an acquired autoimmune disorder, although circulating antibody titres do not correlate well with disease severity. Circulating IgG autoantibodies bind to components of the basement membrane zone of the skin, most commonly to BP230 (within the cellular part of hemidesmosomes) or BP180 (a transmembrane molecule).
Complement is then activated, an inflammatory cascade starts, and mast cells liberate their content of inflammatory mediators. The possibility of an association with internal malignancy remains controversial.

Diagnosis

Differential diagnosis is described in Figure 62.

Biopsy of a new pemphigoid blister shows that it is subepidermal, often with an inflammatory infiltrate containing eosinophils. Direct immunofluorescence, best performed on non-blistered skin, shows a linear band of IgG and C3 along the basement membrane.

Treatment[1]

Fig. 62. Differential diagnosis of pemphigoid.

The aim is to suppress the eruption, without causing side-effects, until spontaneous remission occurs. However, so far, the evidence favouring

Pemphigoid: differential diagnosis	
Eczema/urticaria	Pemphigoid sometimes starts with a pre-bullous stage rather like eczema or urticaria.
Pemphigus	No urticarial background, prominent mouth involvement, blisters rupture more easily leaving erosions.
Cicatricial pemphigoid	Occasionally has a generalized eruption like that of pemphigoid, but the emphasis is on scarring lesions of mucous membranes.
Dermatitis herpetiformis, linear IgA disease, the acquired type of epidermolysis bullosa, and erythema multiforme	Can look like pemphigoid but will be separated from it by the test results.

any particular treatment has been based on a handful of randomized clinical trials, involving few patients.[2]

In the past, the mainstay of treatment has been systemic corticosteroids, often with the addition of a steroid-sparing agent, such as azathioprine. This may change now, as a large recent trial has shown that treatment with highly potent topical corticosteroids is at least as good as, if not better than using systemic corticosteroids. Surprisingly, the benefits of topical treatment were especially clear-cut in those with extensive disease.[3]

Future developments

The trend may now be towards topical treatment with highly potent corticosteroids, perhaps supplemented by oral tetracycline, with or without niacinamide.[3]

66The trend may now be towards topical treatment with highly potent corticosteroids 99

PHOTOSENSITIVITY

Introduction

The skin is our main defence against light, and in particular against ultraviolet (UV) radiation. Sometimes the skin reacts abnormally to light by becoming inflamed. This is *photosensitivity.*

Aetiology

There are many causes of photosensitivity. Some of the most important are listed in Figure 63. These reactions are either a direct toxic effect of light, or have an immunological component, either provoked by light alone or in conjunction with something else, such as a drug.

Diagnosis and treatment of common causes of photosensitivity[1]

Sunburn

The acute effects of sun on the skin are all too familiar. They are caused largely by medium wavelength UV radiation (UVB), but the "dose" required to produce sunburn depends on:

- An individual's skin type (Figure 64).
- The intensity of the radiation (greatest near the equator and around midday).
- The length of exposure to UVB.

Mild sunburn causes erythema: more severe damage leads to extensive blistering and epidermal loss.

66 Caused largely by medium wavelength UV radiation (UVB) 99

Fig. 63. Some important causes of photosensitivity.

Acute
- Sunburn
- Xeroderma pigmentosum
- Porphyria
- Solar urticaria
- Pellagra

Important causes of photosensitivity

Photosensitivity disorders
- Polymorphic light eruption
- Juvenile spring eruption
- Hydroa vacciniforme
- Actinic prurigo

Disorders exacerbated by light
- Drug reactions
- Lupus erythematosus
- Rosacea
- Darier's disease
- Eczema (including actinic dermatitis and photocontact dermatitis)
- Psoriasis
- Lichen planus

Fig. 64. Susceptibility of different skin types to sunburn.

Skin type	
Type I	Always burns, never tans
Type II	Burns easily, tans poorly
Type III	Burns occasionally, tans well
Type IV	Never burns, tans well
Type V	Genetically "brown" (for example, Asian skin)
Type VI	Genetically "black" (for example, African/Caribbean skin)

Treatment

Treatment makes little difference to the acute changes, but symptomatic relief can be obtained with soothing lotions, such as calamine.

Preventive measures

These include avoiding the midday sun, seeking shade, wearing appropriate clothing and eyewear, and using sunscreens. This is more important for those with skin types I and II than for those with a more resilient skin.

Porphyria

Some forms of porphyria are associated with photosensitivity. In a European child the most common is erythropoietic protoporphyria, whereas an adult presenting for the first time probably has porphyria cutanea tarda. The latter is often associated with alcoholic liver disease. Screening tests involve blood, urine and stool samples and are best undertaken in a specialist setting.

❝Porphyria cutanea tarda is often associated with alcoholic liver disease ❞

Solar urticaria

Rarely, exposure to light leads to urticarial weals.

Pellagra

In Western societies, nicotinic acid deficiency is seen most commonly in alcoholics. It presents a triad of changes:

- Diarrhoea
- Dementia
- Dermatitis, which is light sensitive

Polymorphic light eruption

This is perhaps the most important, and certainly the commonest of the primary photosensitivity disorders. Patients often refer to their skin changes as "prickly heat", but true prickly heat (or miliaria rubra) is quite different.

❝Prickly heat is quite different ❞

Polymorphic light eruption presents a day or two after sun exposure, with changes on light exposed areas, for example the forearms, legs, the "V" of the neck and the face. The lesions are itchy and morphologically variable (hence "polymorphic"). There may be papules, plaques, blisters or areas resembling eczema (Figure 65). They increase in intensity over a week or so before subsiding.

Treatment

Treatment with topical steroids provides some relief, but some patients require systemic steroids to control an acute attack.

Fig. 65. An example of a photosensitive dermatosis: polymorphic light eruption on the back of the hand and wrist.

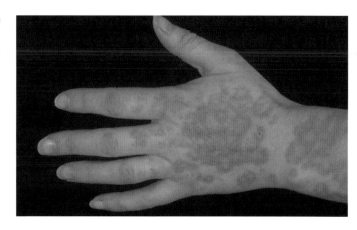

Prevention

Prevention is a better approach. Unfortunately, sunscreens are often not effective, but pre-season PUVA works well and can last for a whole summer. An alternative is the use of antimalarial medication (notably hydroxychloroquine) taken during sunny periods, or while abroad.

A variant of polymorphic light eruption (*juvenile spring eruption*) occurs almost exclusively in boys. Clusters of small blisters appear on the tops of the ears, especially in early spring. The condition settles spontaneously with age.

66 A variant of polymorphic light eruption (juvenile spring eruption) occurs almost exclusively in boys 99

Hydroa vacciniforme

This is rare. It presents in childhood with blistering on the face after sun exposure. The lesions heal to leave scars.

Disorders exacerbated by light

* Some drugs, notably phenothiazines, sulphonamides and thiazides may be associated with reactions to UV.
* The rash of acute systemic lupus erythematosus is classically photosensitive.
* The lesions of chronic discoid lupus erythematosus are also often worse after sun exposure.
* Psoriasis and lichen planus can both be exacerbated by light.
* Patients with rosacea frequently report deterioration after exposure to sunlight, as do a number of patients with eczema.

However, there are two more specific situations in which light causes eczematous skin changes:

* Actinic dermatitis. Eczematous changes appear on light-exposed areas, notably the face. These become fixed and fluctuate only to a limited extent with the seasons.

- Photocontact dermatitis. Exposure to some chemicals plus UV radiation can induce both phototoxic and photoallergic reactions, most often seen on the backs of the hands and forearms, and on the face.

PITYRIASIS VERSICOLOR

Introduction
The term "versicolor" is a good one and refers to the way that lesions change colour after exposure to sunlight. The name "tinea versicolor" has now been dropped because this is not a dermatophyte infection. Switching to "pityriasis" (Greek for a branny type of scaling) is only a slight improvement.

Definition
The affected areas are fawn or pink against an untanned white skin. They have a characteristic fine surface wrinkling and scaling, and are mainly on the trunk. After exposure to the sun, the areas turn pale and stand out against the tanned background.

"The affected areas are fawn or pink against an untanned white skin"

Aetiology
Pityriasis versicolor is due to the overgrowth of skin yeasts (Malassezia species), which are part of the normal skin flora. When stimulated by ultraviolet light they release carboxylic acids that inhibit local melanogenesis.
Predisposing factors include:
- Age: oily skin – peak in early 20s
- A hot climate
- Systemic corticosteroids (or Cushing's disease)

"Pityriasis versicolor is due to the overgrowth of skin yeasts"

Diagnosis
Microscopy of scrapings reveals a "spaghetti and meatballs" appearance as the mycelial form of the organism predominates over yeast-like forms. Culture is a waste of time as these yeasts are found on everyone's skin.

The main diagnostic difficulty is telling the non-scaly pale areas of treated versicolor from vitiligo (larger lesions, more completely depigmented, often affects the face and limbs). Seborrhoeic dermatitis (more inflamed, presternal and interscapular distribution) comes into the differential diagnosis of darker lesions.

"Microscopy of scrapings reveals a "spaghetti and meatballs" appearance"

Treatment
The main problem with topical treatment is applying it over such wide areas, hence the vogue for lathering on shampoos containing an

anti-yeast element (for example, ketoconazole or selenium sulphide). Recommended regimens vary, from applications being left on overnight to washing them off after 10 minutes, and from use on alternate days for 2 to 4 weeks to just 1 or 2 applications. Relapse rates are high.

66Systemic itraconazole is effective 99

Systemic itraconazole is effective. A single dose of 400mg may be as good as 200mg daily for 7 days.[1] Most reserve it for widespread or stubborn eruptions, others recommend it routinely. Using shampoo treatment monthly for the next few months reduces the risk of relapse.

Patients must be warned in advance that none of these treatments will bring their pigment back immediately; this takes many months.

Fig. 66. The pathways involved in the sensation of itching.

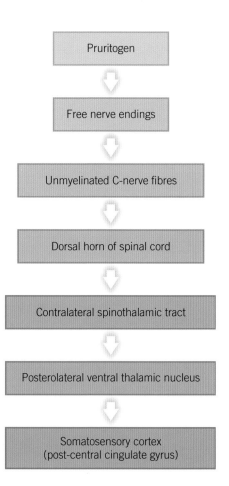

Action	Agent
Direct stimulation of itch-specific C-fibres	Histamine Papain Kallikrein Interleukin-2 Acetyl choline (only in atopy)
Via histamine release	Chymase Trypsin Vasoactive intestinal peptide Substance P Serotonin Bradykinin
Potentiate the action of histamine but with no pruritogenic action of their own	Prostaglandins

Fig. 67. Some pruritogens and their mode of action.

PRURITUS (GENERALIZED)

Introduction

Acute itch may have a useful protective function. Chronic itch is usually a nuisance, and the most unpleasant symptom of many skin diseases. It also has a variety of internal causes that may need to be investigated.

Definition

Itching is like an elephant: easy to recognize but hard to define. The classical definition is "an unpleasant sensation that provokes the desire to scratch" and, although circular, it has survived since 1660 despite attempts to replace it.[1]

Aetiology

The itch pathway[2] is shown in Figure 66. Many endogenous chemicals cause itching when injected into the skin, some by releasing histamine (Figure 67). In addition, itching can follow damage to its neurological pathways, for example from multiple sclerosis.

***Itching can follow damage to its neurological pathways**￼*

Diagnosis

One approach to this difficult problem is given in Figure 68.

81

Diagnostic step	Example
Step 1. Decide if the itching is caused by a skin disorder. Sometimes these can be subtle and hard to identify.	Common examples include: 1. Dry skin in the elderly 2. Scabies in the cleanly 3. Low-grade but widespread atopic eczema 4. Excoriated dermatitis herpetiformis 5. Intermittent urticaria or dermographism
Step 2. Consider external causes that do not necessarily cause a rash.	Examples include fibreglass, wool, and low humidity.
Step 3. Next think about internal causes of itching. A full history and physical examination are needed. Any clinical pointers should be followed up.	Examples are given in Figure 69. The presence of a "butterfly sign" suggests an internal cause.
Step 4. If there are still no clues, and an internal cause is still suspected, perform a simple battery of tests. Repeat at intervals if the diagnosis remains obscure.	These might include a full blood count, ESR, plasma creatinine, liver function tests, thyroid function tests, and chest X-ray.

Fig. 68. Diagnostic decisions to be made in generalized pruritus.

Treatment

If a cause for itching is found, treat it. Failing this, symptomatic measures are needed, but are not always effective.

General measures

These are listed in Figure 70.

Topical treatment

- Always try an emollient. This is best applied after a bath or shower because itching is often associated with dry skin, particularly in the elderly. Many emollients are available and patients will select the one they like best by trial and error.
- 1% menthol or phenol in aqueous cream applied twice a day is often helpful.

Group	Examples
Metabolic/endocrine	• Hyper- or hypothyroidism • Renal failure • Cholestasis, including that of pregnancy • Iron deficiency • Carcinoid syndrome • Mastocytosis • Diabetes (rare)
Malignancy	• Mainly lymphomas
Neuropsychiatric	• A few cerebral tumours cause nasal itch • Multiple sclerosis • Depression in the elderly
Drugs	• Opiates, aspirin, gold, drugs causing cholestasis
Others	• HIV infection

Fig. 69. Internal causes of generalized itching with no rash.

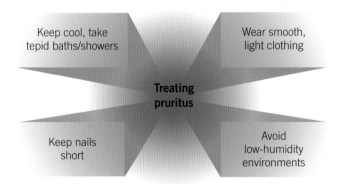

Fig. 70. General measures for treating pruritus.

Keep cool, take tepid baths/showers

Wear smooth, light clothing

Treating pruritus

Keep nails short

Avoid low-humidity environments

- Doxepin cream helps some patients with atopic eczema; topical local anaesthetics and capsaicin can be considered for localized itching.

83

Systemic treatment

- There is no "all-purpose" antipruritic agent.
- Non-sedative H1-receptor antagonists help histamine-mediated itch only. Sometimes there is an added effect if they are combined with an H2-receptor antagonist.
- For non-histamine-mediated itch, a sedative H1-receptor antagonist is worth trying. This works by way of its sedative qualities.
- Doxepine, a tricyclic antidepressant with H1- and H2-receptor antagonist properties, may be worth a trial.
- Other drugs to consider include paroxetine, a serotonin selective reuptake inhibitor, and mirtazapine, an antidepressant with H1 antihistamine properties.

PSORIASIS[1]

Introduction

" A common skin disorder characterized by an increase in the thickness of the epidermis "

Psoriasis is a common skin disorder characterized by an increase in the thickness of the epidermis, alterations in the normal process of keratinization and changes to cutaneous blood vessels. In many, if not all patients, there is genetic susceptibility, although it is not clear how this operates in a particular individual, and what effect the environment has.

Definition and epidemiology

Psoriasis affects 2-3% of most populations, although some ethnic groups (notably Afro-Caribbeans) have a lower prevalence. Ultimately, psoriasis is defined by its histology, which is highly characteristic (Figure 71) and explains the cardinal clinical features of the disease.

Fig. 71. The highly characteristic histology of psoriasis.

The histology of psoriasis

- Epidermal acanthosis (thickening of the prickle cell layer)
- Dilated blood vessels in upper dermis
- Loss of granular cell layer and "parakeratosis" (retention of nuclei in corneocytes)
- Collections of polymorphs in epidermis

Aetiology

The alterations in epidermal organization and growth found in psoriasis seem to be the result of an autoimmune process. The genetic predisposition present in most, if not all, patients is likely to cause this. In addition, external factors can trigger or exacerbate psoriasis. Stress, physical trauma and streptococcal infections are all associated with fresh attacks and the deterioration of existing psoriasis.

What remains completely unknown is why the first lesions of psoriasis appear when they do, and why some areas of the body surface are affected and others are not.

Diagnosis

There are several variants of psoriasis (Figure 72). Their key diagnostic features are described below. Examples are also shown in Figure 73.

Classical plaque

Most patients have a number of slowly evolving scaly red plaques. Histology is occasionally the final arbiter, but the decision that a rash is psoriasis is usually made clinically, based on the characteristics of the lesions and on their distribution. In classical "plaque" psoriasis these are remarkably constant (Figure 74).

“Most patients have a number of slowly evolving scaly red plaques”

Guttate psoriasis

Guttate means "drop-like" and patients with this form are covered in showers of small lesions, each with the same surface characteristics as plaque psoriasis. There may be an accentuation on the extensor sur-

---

Clinical variants of psoriasis

- Classical plaque (psoriasis vulgaris)

- Guttate

- Flexural

- Pustular:
  - acute
  - chronic (of palms and soles)

- Unstable/erythrodermic

- Arthropathic

- Nail

Fig. 72. Clinical variants of psoriasis.

Fig. 73. (a) Typical patches of psoriasis on the elbow. (b) A circumscribed patch of psoriasis on the scalp.

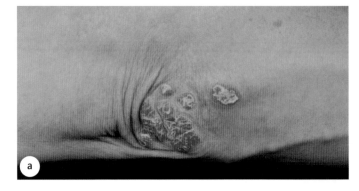

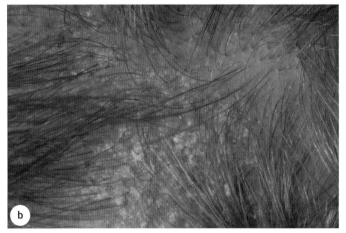

faces too. The condition often appears suddenly with no pre-existing history, or may follow an infection, particularly a streptococcal sore throat. Once established, active guttate psoriasis may not settle, but evolves instead into classical plaques.

Flexural psoriasis

66 It can be difficult to tell flexural psoriasis from seborrhoeic eczema 99

Psoriasis has a predilection for the axillae, infra-mammary folds, natal cleft and groin creases. The rubbing inevitable in such sites removes the surface scales, leaving the lesions red and shiny. It can be difficult to tell flexural psoriasis from seborrhoeic eczema (page 43), although involvement of the natal cleft or umbilicus strongly favours psoriasis. Nail changes are diagnostic.

Pustular psoriasis

There are two different forms of psoriasis in which pustules are prominent:

Fig. 74. Features of plaque psoriasis.

Classic plaque psoriasis

Characteristics of individual lesions

- Fixed, or slowly evolving
- Raised
- Red
- Scaly: scale reflects light; often described as "silvery"
- Gentle scraping of the surface reveals pinpoint bleeding

Distribution/sites of predilection

- Knees
- Elbows
- Scalp
- Base of spine
- Umbilicus

Acute (of von Zumbusch)

The body is covered in sheeted erythema, studded with pustules. Patients are toxic, with a high temperature. Fortunately, this is very rare.

Chronic (of palms and soles)

Waves of pustules appear on patches of erythema and scaling on the palms and soles. There are often no other features of psoriasis. This is common and can be disabling. This type is associated with smoking.

"Chronic type is associated with smoking"

Unstable/erythrodermic psoriasis

Psoriatic lesions can cease to be stable and fixed: instead, they can spread rapidly. As their extent increases, the patches merge into each other, and the ability of the skin to control heat loss is compromised. This state is known as erythroderma or exfoliative dermatitis.

Arthropathic psoriasis

Up to 10% of patients with psoriasis develop a sero-negative, reactive arthropathy. There characteristic patterns are given in Figure 75.

Fig. 75. Patterns of arthropathic psoriasis.

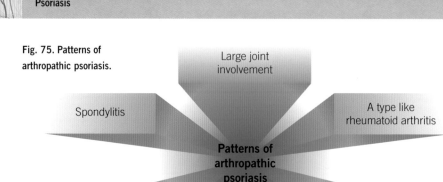

Nail changes

"Nail involvement is one of the most characteristic features of psoriasis"

Nail involvement is one of the most characteristic features of psoriasis. The following changes can occur:

- Pits: these are irregularly distributed and may distort the nail surface.
- Onycholysis: lifting of the nail plate begins distally and spreads towards the nail fold.
- Subungual hyperkeratosis: the area beneath the nail becomes thickened and friable.
- Pustular change: very rarely a nail is virtually destroyed by chronic pustular psoriasis.

Prevention

Nothing can be done to prevent psoriasis occurring *per se*, although avoiding known triggers makes sense. In particular, it is important to be wary of using irritant agents or very potent topical steroids on unstable psoriasis because this can destabilize the situation further.

While apparently logical, there is little evidence that tonsillectomy really does prevent repeated attacks of guttate psoriasis.

Treatment

There are many therapeutic agents with a proven efficacy in psoriasis, but none provides a permanent solution. The choice should be tailored to each individual, and decisions rest on assessing the severity of the disease as perceived by the patient, and the degree to which the patient is prepared to accept risks and inconvenience in the pursuit of relief.

The principal options and their indications are summarized in Figure 76, but the simplest approach is to start with a topical agent and then add or substitute other agents as appropriate.

Therapeutic options in psoriasis	
Emollients	Useful for reducing scale.
Tar	Often used in combination therapies and with UVB. Useful for scalp disease.
Salicylic acid	Often used in combination therapies. Reduces scale.
Dithranol	Safe and effective, but messy and can burn. Undoubtedly successful if patients are prepared for the effort involved.
Vitamin D analogues	Often first-line topical therapy. Should not be overused because of their effects on calcium metabolism.
Topical corticosteroids	Effective short-term and important in scalp disease. Side-effects after chronic use make alternation with other therapies desirable.
Vitamin A analogues: – Topical – Systemic	 Moderately effective in plaque disease. Etretinate used for widespread or severe disease. Teratogenic and may cause hyperlipidaemia.
UVB	Very effective in 70% of patients, if they can make the time to attend hospital. Particularly successful for guttate disease.
PUVA	Very effective combination of UVA and a psoralen, taken systemically, or applied to the skin. The psoralen sensitizes the skin to the effects of the UVA. Used particularly for extensive disease, or for hands and feet. The total lifetime quantity is limited by the risk of skin cancer.
Methotrexate	Weekly tablets can control severe disease. Safer than often thought, although requires careful monitoring.
Ciclosporin	Often dramatically effective but associated with significant side-effects and reserved for severe disease.

Fig. 76. Options for treating psoriasis.

PYOGENIC GRANULOMA

Introduction

Pyogenic granuloma is a misleading term applied to benign lesions that can appear almost anywhere, and can be a considerable nuisance. They are not granulomatous, and their pyogenic (pus-producing) potential is highly variable (Figure 77).

Definition and epidemiology

Pyogenic granulomas are benign masses of vascular granulation tissue. They occur mostly in the young.

Aetiology

Some pyogenic granulomas arise spontaneously: others follow minor trauma or an inflammatory lesion, such as an acne spot.

Diagnosis

66Most common on digits, and on the head and neck 99

Lesions arise rapidly, often over a few days. They can occur anywhere but are most common on digits, and on the head and neck. Most, at least early in their course, are polypoid. They often have a narrow base, with a "collar". They bleed profusely on contact. As lesions mature, the surface epithelializes and the bleeding tendency diminishes. Some disappear completely if left alone.

It can be hard to be sure that a pyogenic granuloma is not something more sinister, particularly in an older person. It is therefore good practice to obtain histology if there is any doubt about the diagnosis.

Fig. 77. Pyogenic granuloma: a juicy, but benign tumour.

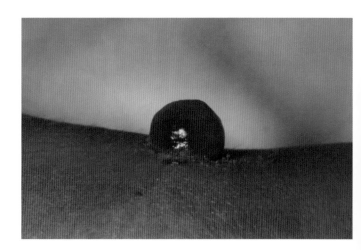

Treatment

Treatment may be with cryotherapy, using liquid nitrogen, but this is not always effective and can lead to considerable bleeding. The authors prefer to curette suspected pyogenic granulomas, cauterizing the base (which may bleed profusely) carefully. This has the advantage of allowing the specimen to be examined histologically. Occasionally pyogenic granulomas recur.

ROSACEA

Introduction and background

The term "acne rosacea" has, rightly, been dropped. Rosacea is not a type of acne. Similarly, old ideas about rosacea being caused by an excessive intake of tea, or chronic embarrassment, have been disproved.

Definition and epidemiology[1]

The lesions of rosacea are erythematous papules and pustules set symmetrically against a background of erythema and telangiectasia over the cheeks, chin, forehead and nose (Figure 78). Sufferers from rosacea flush easily and often, sometimes with a burning sensation. Rosacea is common in middle-aged adults, especially fair-skinned ones. Women are affected more often than men.

"Sufferers from rosacea flush easily"

Aetiology

This remains unclear. The ideas that rosacea is an extra-gastric manifestation of a *Helicobacter pylori* infection,[2] or related to a multiplication of *Demodex folliculorum* mites, have yet to be proved.

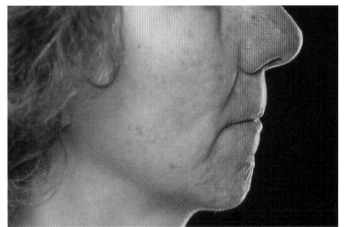

Fig. 78. Typical facial rosacea with early rhinophyma.

Fig. 79. Factors that make rosacea worse.

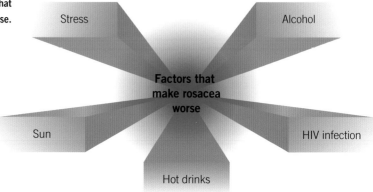

Some factors that make rosacea worse are shown in Figure 79. Complications include:

- Psychological problems (loss of confidence and anxiety, leading to depression).
- Eye involvement (rosacea keratitis in 5%, irritable eyes in many more. Oral and topical antibiotics are helpful. The severity of eye involvement does not correlate with that of the skin lesions).
- Chronic lymphoedema of the face (sometimes helped by massage).
- Rebound flares if corticosteroids are used and then stopped.
- Rhinophyma (a bulbous overgrowth of nasal sebaceous glands).

Diagnosis

This is made on clinical grounds. Unlike acne, rosacea has no comedones, but has a background of erythema, and affects the central face. Seborrhoeic dermatitis lacks papules and pustules. The flushing of rosacea is occasionally confused with that of the menopause or carcinoid.

Treatment

This is empirical because the cause of rosacea is still not understood. Known trigger factors should be avoided. Topical metronidazole formulations help mild-to-moderate rosacea. Other topical possibilities include clindamycin lotion, permethrin cream, and azaleic acid.

For more severe rosacea, topical treatments can be combined with an oral antibiotic (usually tetracycline or oxytetracycline, or erythromycin at 500mg twice a day for 6 to 12 weeks). Oral metronidazole is also effective but carries the risks of mutagenicity and of peripheral neuropathy. Topical metronidazole often keeps patients in remission after oral antibiotics have been stopped.

❝ Topical metronidazole often keeps patients in remission after oral antibiotics ❞

Other treatments include:

- Cosmetic camouflage
- Medication to reduce flushing (clonidine or a beta blocker)
- A vascular laser for telangiectasia
- Plastic surgery for rhinophyma[3]
- Oral isotretinoin, occasionally, for severe and refractory cases

Future developments

There are encouraging reports of the value of treatments to eradicate *H. pylori*. Topical tacrolimus may also be beneficial.

SCABIES

Introduction and background

There are many effective treatments for scabies (Figure 80), but it still flourishes as it has done for centuries. Its diagnosis and treatment are easy in theory but not in practice, and its prevalence fluctuates wildly for reasons that are not fully understood.

Diagnostic errors are still made in about 25% of cases, and this rises when scabies is uncommon and doctors are less familiar with it. In addition, those who have scabies are not known for the meticulous way in which they follow treatment, and often become reinfested from unmentioned and untreated contacts.

❝Diagnostic errors are still made in about 25% of cases, and this rises when scabies is uncommon and doctors are less familiar with it❞

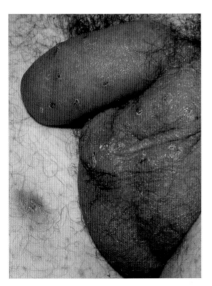

Fig. 80. These excoriated scrotal nodules can only be due to scabies. Reproduced with kind permission from Savin JA, Junter JA and Hepburn N. Diagnosis in Color: Skin Signs in Clinical Medicine. London: Mosby Ltd, 1997.

Definition and epidemiology

66 *Overcrowding, poor hygiene and poverty are associated* 99

Overcrowding, poor hygiene and poverty are associated with high levels of scabies, which is caused by the mite *Sarcoptes scabiei* var. hominis. High levels are constant in under-developed countries, whereas in richer countries prevalence rates fluctuate strikingly at intervals varying from 10 to 20 years.

Two rival theories have been advanced to explain these peaks of prevalence. The first ties them to social unrest, and examples have been seen after civil disasters and during World Wars. The second suggests that "herd immunity" builds up during an epidemic, so that the next one can appear only when a new and susceptible generation has arisen.

Aetiology

Scabies and its mites have these characteristics:

- Adult female mites are about 0.4mm long and can just be seen through a lens. Adult males are about half as long and seldom found.
- Mites spread from person to person through prolonged bodily contact rather than via inanimate objects.
- Patients with scabies host an average of 12 adult female mites, which lay about 40 to 50 eggs in a burrow during their life span of 4 to 6 weeks. In unworn clothing, they die in about a week.
- Mites move over warm skin at up to 2.5cm a minute, but burrow through the stratum corneum at only about 2mm a day, sticking mainly to areas with relatively few hair follicles.

Fig. 81. Differential diagnosis of scabies.

Condition	Clinical pointers
Animal scabies	An itchy pet. The rash of the owner looks like scabies but lacks burrows
Papular urticaria (reactions to insect bites)	Excoriated papules in lines or groups
Low-grade, late onset atopic eczema	No burrows; a history of atopy
Fibreglass itching	History of contact
Others to consider	Lichen planus, neurotic excoriations, dermatitis herpetiformis

- Itching takes 3 to 5 weeks to appear in a first infestation, but only a few days in subsequent ones.
- Mites are found most easily in burrows, and the widespread eruption and generalized itching are due to allergy to the mite and its products.

Diagnosis

The differential diagnosis is given in Figure 81.

Pointers towards a diagnosis of scabies include:
- Itching that is worse at night.
- Friends and family members who are also itchy.
- Burrows are pathognomonic. Most lie on the finger webs and on the sides of the fingers, wrists and hands. Other favourite sites include the feet, nipples, genitals and elbows.
- On the genitals, burrows appear as erythematous nodules, which may persist long after the infestation has cleared.
- The face is affected only in infants.

The best proof of the diagnosis is to find an acarus. There are several ways of doing this. An experienced clinician can usually pick one out neatly with a needle, from the newest, least scaly end of a burrow. Alternatively, mites and eggs can be seen microscopically in burrow scrapings mounted in potassium hydroxide or mineral oil. Dermatoscopy, with or without a video,[1] is gaining popularity as a quick and easy way to detect acari.

> **The best proof of the diagnosis is to find an acarus**

Prevention

Outbreaks in hospitals or residential homes can sometimes be solved by finding a patient with "crusted" (also known as "Norwegian") scabies. This is seen in mentally handicapped, demented or paralysed patients, or in the immunosuppressed.

Crusted, almost warty areas appear on the hands and feet, nails thicken, and a widespread erythema completes the picture. Scrapings from all areas show huge numbers of mites and eggs. Itching can be minimal, and undiagnosed cases are often responsible for outbreaks of scabies.

Treatment with ivermectin is needed (see below), combined with topical measures. Patients with "crusted" scabies should be isolated until they are clear, and their clothing and bedding should be laundered.[2]

> **Patients with "crusted" scabies should be isolated**

Treatment[3,4,5]

This has changed in several ways over the last few years. It is no longer recommended that a hot bath should be taken before using topical treatments as this may increase their absorption. Treatment should be applied to the scalp, neck, face and ears as well as to the rest of the body surface. Particular attention should be paid to finger webs and the lotion should be brushed under nails.

"Malathion and permethrin are now the topical treatments of choice in the UK"

Malathion and permethrin are now the topical treatments of choice in the UK, preferably as aqueous rather than alcoholic solutions. Both need two applications, one week apart. Older and less effective preparations include benzyl benzoate, which may need up to three applications on consecutive days.

Ivermectin (as a single oral dose of 200mg/kg body weight) is effective. A second dose, taken 7–10 days later, improves the cure rate. This suggests that the drug may not be active at all stages in the life cycle of the parasite.[6] It is available in the UK on a named patient basis, and worth considering, with local treatment, for "crusted" scabies. Its safety in pregnant women and young children has yet to be established.

The following principles remain unchanged:

- Give patients a printed treatment sheet, and go through it with them in detail.
- Make sure they understand that treatment must be applied to all areas and not just to the itchy parts of the skin.
- Secondary infection is common, but not a reason for postponing scabies treatment. Superadded bacterial infection should be treated on its own merits, bearing in mind that it can sometimes trigger glomerulonephritis.
- Pay more attention to the patients than to their clothing and bedding. Ordinary laundering will cope with these.

"Treat all family members and sexual contacts"

- Treat all family members and sexual contacts, whether itchy or not: reinfestation inevitably follows failure to do this.
- Itching often continues after treatment. Crotamiton or calamine applications, and possibly a sedating antihistamine at night, should deal with this.
- Take special care with pregnant or lactating women and very young children, as evidence on treatment safety is weak. Old-fashioned remedies, such as 6% sulphur in soft white paraffin, or 25% benzyl benzoate emulsion diluted with three parts of water, may be worth considering.
- Screen adults with scabies for sexually transmitted diseases that can be picked up at the same time.

Future developments

Treatment is easier to use if it is oral rather than topical. Oral ivermectin may yet be used routinely to treat individuals with scabies, and as a prophylactic for their close contacts. Attempts could even be made to eradicate endemic scabies from areas where its prevalence is high.[7] However, the risk of resistance developing must always be kept in mind.

SEBORRHOEIC KERATOSIS

Introduction

The commonest benign tumours of human skin are seborrhoeic keratoses (*seborrhoeic warts, senile warts, basal cell papillomas*). Their main importance lies in their nuisance value – they can be itchy, sore and unsightly – and in the need to separate them from more threatening lesions, especially malignancies.

Definition and epidemiology

Seborrhoeic warts have a characteristic histology. They are extremely common, particularly in older people. Some patients have a strong family history of the condition, suggesting a genetic predisposition.

Aetiology

Seborrhoeic warts are usually age-related, although as indicated above, there may be genetic influences. Very rarely, masses of itchy seborrhoeic warts develop rapidly in association with an internal malignancy (the sign of Leser and Trélat).

Diagnosis

Lesions can appear anywhere but are most common on the trunk and the head and neck. Most are unmistakable, showing a "stuck-on" appearance (Figure 82). Their surface is often said to be "greasy," but "grainy" may be a better description, with small pseudo-follicular dents and protrusions. The colour ranges from pale pink, through shades of brown, to jet-black.

Usually a clinical diagnosis is sufficient, but very dark seborrhoeic warts can give rise to genuine difficulty in distinguishing them clinically

> *Most are unmistakable, showing a "stuck-on" appearance*

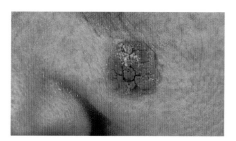

Fig. 82. A typical seborrhoeic keratosis.
Reproduced with kind permission from Graham-Brown R and Bourke JF. Mosby's Colour Atlas and Text of Dermatology. London: Mosby Ltd, 1999.

97

from a malignant melanoma. Occasionally, similar doubts about malignancy can be thrown up by a seborrhoeic wart that becomes inflamed or bleeds. If there is doubt, excision for histology is simple and diagnostic.

Treatment

If treatment is needed, cryotherapy with liquid nitrogen is probably the best approach

Many lesions require no treatment. Some are symptomatic (itch, soreness, catching on clothing, bleeding) and patients often request others to be removed on cosmetic grounds. If there is no doubt about the diagnosis and treatment is needed, cryotherapy with liquid nitrogen is probably the best approach. An alternative is curettage and cautery. Very large lesions may be best excised formally.

SQUAMOUS CELL CARCINOMA

Introduction[1]

A squamous cell carcinoma is a primary malignancy of the epidermis. It can, and does, metastasize. Lesions around and on mucosal surfaces are likely to spread earlier and more extensively than those on "ordinary" skin.

Definition and epidemiology

Squamous cell carcinoma is an invasive malignancy of epidermal keratinocytes with the capacity to metastasize.

Aetiology

More common with age and cumulative sun exposure

Squamous cell carcinoma becomes gradually more common with age and cumulative sun exposure. Immunosuppression, especially in transplant patients,[2,3] is an increasing issue as patients now live longer and can spend more time out-of-doors. UVB, and especially PUVA, used to treat skin diseases are other risk factors. Infection with the human papilloma virus is implicated in some squamous cell carcinomas, especially of the genitalia.

Diagnosis

The features of cutaneous squamous cell carcinomas range from small, indolent scabs, to deep, rapidly growing ulcers (Figure 83). Any persistent, enlarging, keratotic or ulcerative lesion on light-exposed skin should be considered suspicious. A biopsy is mandatory. Ideally excision should be undertaken immediately.

Under current Department of Health standards, any lesion suspected of being a squamous cell carcinoma should be seen in a specialist unit within 2 weeks.

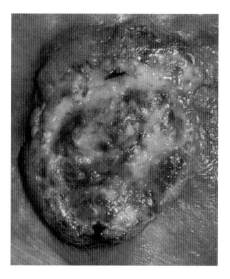

Fig. 83. A poorly differentiated squamous cell carcinoma. Reproduced with kind permission from Graham-Brown R and Bourke JF. Mosby's Colour Atlas and Text of Dermatology. London: Mosby Ltd, 1999.

Prevention

Avoiding excessive sun exposure is crucial, especially for those at high risk, for example those on post-transplant immunosuppression.

Treatment[4]

The most effective treatment is adequate excision of the primary tumour. Radiotherapy helps large, or awkward lesions, especially in the very old. Follow-up treatments for recurrences or spread are the province of specialist multi-disciplinary teams.

❝ The most effective treatment is adequate excision of the primary tumour ❞

URTICARIA AND ANGIO-OEDEMA

Introduction and background

Urticaria is the clinical manifestation of mast cells degranulating in the dermis. In angio-oedema this takes place in the subcutaneous tissues. Often the two occur together. Both are reaction patterns with many causes, not diseases in their own right. In the past this has caused confusion, with physical causes frequently being ignored and allergic ones over-emphasized and over-investigated. Patients like this, but the yields are small.

Fig. 84. Symptomatic dermographism: linear weals at the site of scratching. Reproduced with kind permission from Graham-Brown R and Bourke JF. Mosby's Colour Atlas and Text of Dermatology. London: Mosby Ltd, 1999.

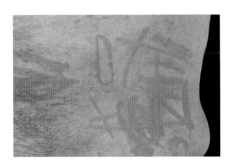

Definition and epidemiology

"Angio-oedema is most common on the lips, eyelids and genitals, and most dangerous in the larynx"

Urticarial weals are transient itchy erythematous swellings, occurring anywhere on the skin (Figure 84). Angio-oedema is most common on the lips, eyelids and genitals, and most dangerous in the larynx.

An individual urticarial lesion usually lasts less than 24 hours before fading to leave no trace. However, new lesions can continue to appear for weeks, months, or even years. By definition, chronic (as opposed to acute) urticaria lasts more than 6 weeks. Only half the patients with chronic urticaria, but without angio-oedema, will be clear in 6 months.

Urticaria is common but often unreported, so its true incidence is hard to assess. Perhaps about 20% of the population have at least one episode of urticaria during their life.

Aetiology

Mast cells can be made to release their contents in many ways. This forms the basis of the classification of urticaria (Figure 85).

The chemicals released include histamine, of course, but also a range of other inflammatory mediators. This is why antihistamines do not always suppress urticaria completely. Once these substances have been released, the local capillaries react by leaking plasma, and weals appear.

Diagnosis

The diagnosis of urticaria falls into two halves.

Type	Subtype	Comment
"Ordinary" urticaria	Acute Chronic	See Figure 86.
Physical urticarias		Can reliably be induced by the same physical stimulus. This forms the basis for appropriate testing. For example, with an ice block. Weals usually last for less than one hour.
	Aquagenic urticaria	Rare. Induced by contact with water.
	Cholinergic urticaria	Small, itchy, transient weals, with surrounding areas of erythema. A response to anxiety, heat, exertion. Avoid heat and excessive exercise. Consider anticholinergics, antihistamines, tranquillizers.
	Cold urticaria	Rare, but warn about the dangers of swimming in cold water. Avoid cold, use protective clothing, antihistamines.
	Delayed pressure urticaria	Lesions slow to appear (after 4–6 hours) and are deep. May affect the soles or palms. Can incapacitate manual workers. Respond poorly to antihistamines.
	Immediate pressure urticaria (dermographism)	Common, may be lifelong or acquired. Lesions are linear. Rubbing the skin reveals exaggeration of the normal "triple response". Avoid friction, use antihistamines if symptomatic
	Localized heat urticaria	Rare. Avoid cause.
	Vibratory angio-oedema	Rare. Avoid cause.
	Solar	Rare. A few have erythropoetic protoporphyria. Avoid sun exposure, use protective clothing, sunscreens, antihistamines.
Angio-oedema without weals		Worth screening for hereditary and acquired C1 esterase inhibitor deficiency. Responds poorly to antihistamines and steroids. Consider long-term use of anabolic steroids.
Contact urticaria		Most often around the mouth in response to foods. Latex is another cause. Avoid cause.
Urticarial vasculitis		Leaves bruised areas. Diagnosis made by biopsy.

Fig. 85. The clinical classification of urticaria and angio-oedema.

Is this really urticaria?

Usually this is obvious, but other possibilities are worth considering. Papular urticaria is a bad term for insect bites. The lesions last longer and are often in groups or lines. Erythema multiforme has characteristic "target lesions". Sometimes the pre-bullous, erythematous phase of pemphigoid causes confusion. Urticarial vasculitis differs from ordinary urticaria in that subsiding lesions leave bruised areas. Some drug eruptions have an urticarial element.

If this is urticaria, which type is it?

This has to be solved clinically, not through the laboratory, on the basis of a detailed history.[1] Physical urticarias are often unrecognized, although they make up about 20% of all urticarias. Think about them particularly if individual weals last for an hour or less. Physical urticarias can often be reproduced by simple tests, for example rubbing brings out dermographism. These are best carried out several days after antihistamines have been stopped.

It is often hard to find an underlying cause for "ordinary" urticarias (see Figure 86). Always ask about drugs (see Figure 87) including self-prescribed ones and herbal medicines.

❝ Testing to suspected allergens may be helpful ❞

The cause of acute urticaria is sometimes obvious, such as an IgE-mediated reaction to a food or a drug. If so, when the episode has settled, radioallergosorbent (RAST) testing or prick testing to suspected allergens (but only if appropriate resuscitation facilities are available) may be helpful. The proven cause, for example peanuts, can then be avoided.

Fig. 86. The causes of "ordinary" urticaria and angio-oedema.

"Ordinary" urticaria and angio-oedema		
Type	**Cause**	**Comment**
Immunological	Autoimmune	Autoantibodies degranulate mast cells by binding to high-affinity IgE receptors or to IgE bound to them
	IgE-dependent	Type 1 hypersensitivity reactions
	Complement-dependent	C1 esterase deficiency
Non-immunological	Drugs, food additives	(See Figure 87)

Drug causes of urticaria	
Drug	**Comment**
Aspirin, NSAIDs and opiates	Aggravate urticaria by non-immunological mechanisms
Penicillin	Usually causes acute urticaria: rarely chronic urticaria is due to its presence in milk
ACE inhibitors	Can cause angio-oedema and aggravate urticaria

Fig. 87. Some drug causes of urticaria.

For chronic urticaria things are seldom as easy, and eventually investigations may be necessary. These should not be routine for all patients, but guided by the history and examination. Mild cases, well controlled by antihistamines do not need to be investigated. Screening tests for non-responders might include a selection of:

• Full blood count
• ESR
• Routine biochemical screen
• Urinalysis
• Thyroid function tests (rarely)
• Autoantibodies (rarely)

Urticaria is seldom due to an underlying disorder, although cases have been seen in infections, intestinal parasitosis, connective tissue disorders and hyperthyroidism.

There is no routine test for histamine-releasing autoantibodies, and no need to perform multiple RAST or skin prick tests. Attempts to correlate clinical state with diet, either by keeping a food diary or by challenge, are time-consuming and poorly rewarded.

Many physical urticarias can be reproduced by appropriate physical tests. Serum C1 esterase inhibitor and C4 levels should be checked in patients with recurrent episodes of angio-oedema without urticaria, and possibly, therefore, in the hereditary type of angio-oedema.

Treatment[2]
General measures
The most important measure is to avoid the underlying cause if this has been established. Failing that, non-specific aggravating factors such as overheating, stress and alcohol should be avoided. Cooling applications (for example, 1% menthol in aqueous cream, or calamine lotion) may help.

"Aggravating factors such as overheating, stress and alcohol should be avoided"

103

Aspirin and NSAIDs must not be taken: paracetamol can be used instead. ACE inhibitors should be used with caution in patients who already have urticaria or angio-oedema.

Treatment of physical urticarias

These are outlined in Figure 85.

Treatment of chronic urticaria

The first-line of treatment is to use a non-sedating H1-blocking antihistamine

The first-line of treatment is to use a non-sedating H1-blocking antihistamine, most of which (except acrivastine) are long acting. The response is usually good.[3] However, mizolastine is contraindicated in heart failure and when the Q-T interval is prolonged, and should not be given at the same time as drugs that can cause cardiac arrhythmia (for example, tricyclic antidepressants) or those that inhibit liver metabolism via cytochrome P450 (for example, macrolide antibiotics and imidazole antifungals).

Patients differ in their response to non-sedating antihistamines. Therefore, if one is not helping, it is worth trying another. Doses can be timed to exert their greatest effect when the urticaria is most active. Sedating antihistamines are seldom used alone now, but can be added to the regimen at night (for example, chlorpheniramine 4-12mg or hydroxyzine 10-50mg) to help an itchy patient sleep better.

Many antihistamines pass into breast milk

Antihistamines should be avoided if possible in pregnancy, especially during the first 3 months. However, if one is needed chlorpheniramine or diphenhydramine are reasonable choices because of their long record of safety. Many antihistamines pass into breast milk.

Other medication

Sometimes using an H2-blocking antihistamine, such as cimetidine, as well as an H1-blocking antihistamine is beneficial. A sympathomimetic agent such as terbutaline may also be effective. Mast-cell stabilizing drugs (for example, ketotifen and nifedipine) are seldom of value. Long-term oral corticosteroids should be avoided in chronic urticaria, although short tapering courses may help acute urticaria, when the cause is known, and severe urticarial vasculitis.

Adrenaline is the appropriate emergency treatment for laryngeal angio-oedema

Adrenaline

This is the appropriate emergency treatment for laryngeal angio-oedema. An intramuscular dose of 500mg (0.5mL adrenaline injection 1 in 1000) is given and can be repeated after an interval if necessary. Adjunctive measures include oxygen and slow intravenous injection of an antihistamine (for example, chlorpheniramine 10-20mg).

Those with severe allergy, at high risk of anaphylaxis or laryngeal oedema, should be taught how to inject adrenaline themselves and should always carry a prefilled adrenaline syringe, such as an Epipen. Unfortunately, adrenaline is not effective for laryngeal oedema of the hereditary type, due to C1 esterase inhibitor deficiency.

66 Adrenaline is not effective for laryngeal oedema of the hereditary type 99

Other interventions
The value of diets free of substances such as tartrazine and salicylates remains controversial.

Future developments
Research is under way on the use of intravenous immunoglobulin and cyclosporin A for severe and unresponsive chronic autoimmune urticaria.

VASCULITIS[1,2]

Introduction
As with other organs, in the skin the blood vessels may be the primary target of disease. The clinical features that follow this are a function of the severity of the damage, and of the size and nature of the vessels involved.

Definition and epidemiology
The term "cutaneous vasculitis" is applied to lesions in which the primary pathological process is vascular inflammation. There is no universally accepted classification. One approach is based on the size of the vessel involved and the type of inflammation – with neutrophils, lymphocytes or granulomas (Figure 88). These are matched with the clinical features (Figure 89).

Aetiology
There are a number of important triggers for cutaneous vasculitis.
- Urticarial vasculitis: lupus erythematosus
- Leucocytoclastic vasculitis (Figure 90): the deposition of immune complexes after a viral or bacterial infection (especially streptococcal) or drug ingestion, paraproteinaemia, autoimmune disorders such as rheumatoid arthritis, and lupus erythematosus
- Perniosis: physical damage from cold
- Erythema nodosum: tuberculosis, sarcoidosis, inflammatory bowel disease, drugs
- Nodular vasculitis: tuberculosis, autoimmune disease, lymphoma
Often no underlying cause can be identified.

Fig. 88. Classification of vasculitits according to size of vessel and type of inflammation.

Classification of vasculitis	
Small vessel	
Urticarial vasculitis	Lymphocytes surround upper dermal vessels
Leucocytoclastic	Neutrophilic inflammation with many fragmented cells and nuclear dust ("leucocytoclasis")
Behçet's disease	Skin lesions are due to a polymorph vasculitis
Chilblains	Cold injury (perniosis) involves lymphocytic vascular damage
Wegener's granulomatosis	Vessels are surrounded by granulomas in this multi-system disorder
Large vessel	
Polyarteritis nodosa	Neutrophilic infiltration affects small- to medium-sized arteries
Vasculitis in lupus erythematosus	Lymphocytes are the predominant cells

Diagnosis

A definitive diagnosis will be based on histology (see Figure 88), but some clinical features are highly suggestive (see Figure 89). Some patients have more than one type of lesion.

Treatment

A full work-up should include screening for autoimmune disease and for paraproteinaemia. If an underlying cause is identified, therapy should be directed at curing or controlling it. Vasculitis of unknown aetiology may respond to dapsone, but some patients require systemic steroids.

❝A full work-up should include screening for autoimmune disease and for para-proteinaemia ❞

Clinical features of vasculitis

Urticarial lesions that persist for more than a few hours and leave a purple stain	Urticarial vasculitis
"Palpable purpura" especially on the lower legs and feet, may appear on extensor surfaces in the Henoch Schönlein syndrome	Leucocytoclastic vasculitis
Deep-seated nodules – on the shins – anywhere	Erythema nodosum Nodular vasculitis
Livedo reticularis	Damage to medium-sized arteries
Ulcers	May occur in various forms and in association with other skin changes

Fig. 89. Clinical features of vasculitis.

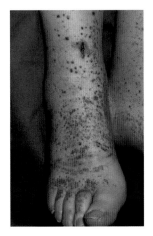

Fig. 90.
Leucocytoclastic
vasculitis on the legs of
an elderly man.
Reproduced with kind
permission from Graham-
Brown R and Bourke JF.
Mosby's Colour Atlas and
Text of Dermatology.
London: Mosby Ltd,
1999.

107

VENOUS ULCERS

Introduction

Leg ulcers are unpleasant and expensive. Treating the nation's leg ulcers takes up about 2% of total health spending in the UK, and the misery they cause more than matches the money spent on them.

Definition and epidemiology

An ulcer is a loss of dermis and epidermis produced by the sloughing of necrotic tissue (Figure 91). At any point in time, 0.1% to 0.2% of the population have one; and this figure rises to 2% in people over 80. Roughly 1% will have a leg ulcer at some time in their lives.

Aetiology

66Venous obstruction, or valvular incompetence, creates superficial venous hypertension and a susceptibility to ulcers 99

Venous obstruction, or valvular incompetence, creates superficial venous hypertension and a susceptibility to ulcers, which are usually triggered by minor trauma.

The features of venous hypertension are:

- At first the legs feel heavy and develop a protein-rich oedema.
- Next they become discoloured red or bluish, sometimes with petechiae and a brown tinge from haemosiderin.
- Later lipodermatosclerosis may appear as an indurated woodiness around the lower leg giving it an "inverted champagne bottle" look.
- Venous ulcers are most common near the medial malleolus.

The underlying factors remain even when an ulcer has healed: hence the common cyclical pattern of healing and recurrence. Recurrence rates of between 40% and 70% are the rule. In addition, other seemingly

Fig. 91. Very severe, chronic ulceration on the lower leg.

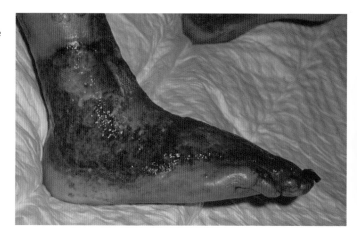

unrelated conditions may be especially common in those with leg ulcers. For example, there is an increased risk of death from ischaemic heart disease.

Factors predisposing to venous ulcers include:
- Deep vein thrombosis
- The presence of varicose veins
- A positive family history

Diagnosis

Venous ulcers favour the gaiter area, and can often be diagnosed by the presence of other signs such as oedema and pigmentation. The differential diagnosis[1] is given in Figure 92.

66 Venous ulcers favour the gaiter area 99

In every case it is important to:
- Look carefully at the edge of the ulcer
- Look at the ulcer bed
- Check the foot pulses
- Check for peripheral neuropathy

Some tests appropriate for a patient with a leg ulcer include:
- A full blood count: anaemia and iron deficiency interfere with healing
- Urine for sugar
- A swab for culture if infection is suspected
- Biopsy if there is suspicion of malignancy

Doppler ankle brachial pressure index: the systolic ankle pressure divided by the systolic brachial pressure. If this is greater than 0.8, the ulcer is unlikely to have an arterial cause.

The other tests selected will depend on the history and clinical findings.

Prevention

After an ulcer has healed, using compression hosiery probably reduces the risk of recurrence. Compliance rates are greater with medium- than high-compression stockings, but patients should be given those with the highest compression they can wear comfortably.

66 Using compression hosiery probably reduces the risk of recurrence 99

Treatment

Expect slow healing if:
- An ulcer is large
- An ulcer has been there a long time
- The patient is immobile
- Oedema and/or anaemia is present

General measures include:
- Losing weight if necessary

- Re-establishing mobility: walking with support bandages does no harm
- Dealing with oedema (diuretics and elevation of the legs for some hours every day)
- Dealing with anaemia
- Using a systemic antibiotic if there is cellulitis or lymphangitis

Fig. 92. Types of non-venous leg ulcer.

Type of ulcer	Clinical points
Due to large vessel arterial disease	Make up 10–20% of all leg ulcers. Punched out, deep, with a pale ulcer bed. More peripheral than venous ulcers. May have rest-pain, claudication, or vascular disease elsewhere. Avoid compression bandaging.
Mixed arterial and venous ulcers	Seen mainly in the elderly. Hard to treat effectively as compression is not possible.
Small vessel disease	Seen in rheumatoid arthritis (10% of sufferers have a leg ulcer at some time), diabetes (foot is the commonest site) and systemic sclerosis.
Pyoderma gangrenosum	Cribriform, with a blue undermined edge. May occur in other areas too. Often accompanied by another disorder such as rheumatoid arthritis, inflammatory bowel disease or paraproteinaemia.
Haematological	Occur in young people. Underlying abnormalities include sickle cell disease, hereditary spherocytosis, and thalassaemia.
Malignant ulcers	Usually a basal or a squamous cell carcinoma. The latter rarely arises in a long-standing venous ulcer. Look for a rolled edge or a heaped up ulcer base, and failure to heal despite treatment.
Neuropathic ulcers	Seen in peripheral neuropathy and diabetes.
Infective	Uncommon in the UK.
Atrophie blanche	A term describing telangiectatic capillaries, seen as pink dots, set against an ivory white background. Ulcers follow minor trauma, and are painful and hard to heal. Can occur with or without venous disease.

Most ulcers can be managed conservatively. Pinch grafting will speed healing if this is clearly going to be very slow. Reviews of the evidence [2,3,4] suggest that:

- Compression increases the rate at which ulcers heal.
- Multilayered systems are more effective than single-layered systems.
- High compression is more effective than low compression but there are no clear differences between the effectiveness of different types of high compression.
- Low adherent dressings are as effective as hydrocolloid dressings beneath compression bandaging.

Many dressings and compression systems are available, the details of which are beyond the scope of this book. The choice depends largely on local preference and expertise. It is important to avoid using compression techniques in ulcers with an arterial component (see use of the Doppler ankle brachial pressure index – Figure 92).

66 Avoid using compression techniques in ulcers with an arterial component 99

VITILIGO

Introduction
Vitiligo is the most important cause of loss of skin pigmentation.

Definition and epidemiology
Vitiligo is an acquired loss of skin colour. Its exact prevalence is unknown, but it is undoubtedly common and often runs in families. It affects adults and children, the latter having the best prognosis. It is not more common or more extensive in dark skin but it is more noticeable and causes more distress. Asian and Afro-Caribbean patients ask for advice especially frequently.

66 Vitiligo is an acquired loss of skin colour 99

Aetiology
Vitiligo is the result of an autoimmune attack on pigment cells (melanocytes). It may occur with other immunological conditions, notably alopecia areata (see page 17). Organ-specific autoantibodies are frequently found.

Diagnosis
Suspect vitiligo when:

- Complete loss of pigment is seen in a patch or patches of skin (Figure 93).
- There has been no prior skin change; in other words, this is not post-inflammatory hypopigmentation.
- There are no other visible or palpable abnormalities.

Fig. 93. A characteristic complete depigmentation with areas of residual pigment in a patch of vitiligo.

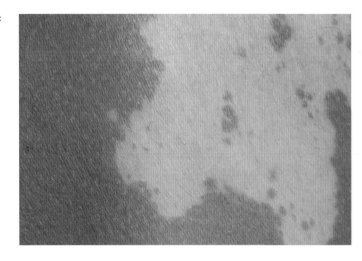

Vitiligo is often symmetrical and is commonly seen around the eyes and mouth, and on the hands, feet and genitalia. If there is darkening around the edge it is called "tri-chrome" vitiligo. The patches usually enlarge slowly, with new areas appearing apparently at random. Some repigment spontaneously and then the skin colour often returns in small dots in the centre of patches.

Prevention

There are no known measures that prevent the onset of vitiligo or stop it worsening, but patients benefit from efforts to camouflage the pale areas. Several ranges of skin-coloured covering agents can make vitiligo invisible and this reduces the psychological effects of the condition.

66The pale patches burn much more quickly than normal skin in the sun 99

The pale patches burn much more quickly than normal skin in the sun. They also become more noticeable if the surrounding areas become tanned. Sunscreens or sun avoidance should be recommended.

Treatment

Success has been claimed for many treatments but few have been supported by good evidence. Topical steroids, used regularly on early lesions, may help, but potent ones are required and carry the risk of side-effects. PUVA can also work and UVB also has its advocates. Whole-body treatment is needed for widespread changes, but local therapy can help limited areas, such as the hands. Topical calcipotriol plus light therapy may be better than light alone.

The long-term steroids and phototherapy do not always produce full repigmentation, but patients are usually pleased with any evidence of improvement.[1]

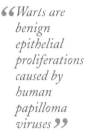

Several other techniques are at a developmental or research stage, for example grafting and various chemicals with or without light.

Occasionally there comes a point where the best option is to depigment the remaining normal skin. In this case a cream containing hydroquinone can be used under specialist supervision.

WARTS (VIRAL)

Definition and epidemiology

Warts are benign epithelial proliferations caused by human papilloma viruses (Figure 94). Common warts occur with increasing frequency during childhood and reach their peak prevalence between age 12 and 16.

❝Warts are benign epithelial proliferations caused by human papilloma viruses❞

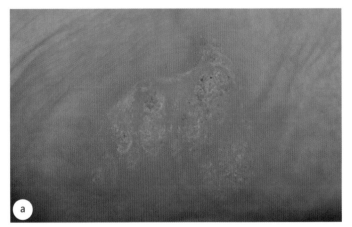

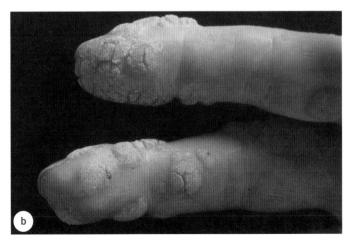

Fig. 94. (a) Verruca on the heel. Thrombosed capillaries can be clearly seen. (b) Very extensive warts on the fingers.

Most warts, therefore, appear in people younger than 20, the exception being anogenital warts, which are most common between 25 and 45.

Aetiology

Human papilloma viruses have been divided into many types by DNA sequencing, but have not yet been cultured *in vitro*. The clinical patterns taken up by warts are determined partly by the genotype of the virus and partly by the site of the infection. Some associations between viral type and presentation are given in Figure 95.

For a wart to appear, virally infected skin scales have had to come into contact with a breach in the skin or mucous membranes – either through direct contact with a wart, or via contaminated objects such as a shower floor with a rough surface. Maceration is a predisposing factor. Incubation times range from 2 to 9 months.

Diagnosis

The diagnosis is made clinically; a biopsy is seldom needed. Some general clinical points to look out for are:

"Black dots of thrombosed vessels differentiate warts from corns and callosities"

- Multiple bleeding points, or the black dots of thrombosed vessels, can be seen when plantar warts are pared: this differentiates them from corns and callosities.
- Warts sometimes follow scratch marks and appear in lines (the Köbner phenomenon). This is especially striking in plane warts.
- Consider an underlying immunodeficiency if warts are unusually numerous, luxuriant or resistant to treatment.
- Consider sexual abuse if children develop anogenital warts. However, most are due to auto-innoculation from warts elsewhere.

Differential diagnosis

The differential diagnoses are described in Figure 96.

Fig. 95. Some associations between clinical pattern and HPV type.

Clinical presentation	Some associated HPV types
Common warts	1, 2, and 4
Plane warts	3 and 10
Genital warts	90% due to 6 and 11 16 and 18 may be oncogenic

Condition	Clinical pointers
Lichen planus	Papules can look like plane warts. Look for Wickham's striae and buccal involvement.
Corns and callosities	No bleeding points seen on paring.
Warty epidermal naevi	Present since birth.
Molluscum contagiosum	Look for characteristic punctum.
Granuloma annulare	Have a smooth surface, often annular.
Syphilis	Condyloma lata are greyer and less well defined than anogenital warts. A blood test will help if there is doubt.
Other lesions to be considered include	Seborrhoeic keratoses, actinic keratoses, cellular naevi, skin tags. All usually spotted easily.

Fig. 96. The differential diagnosis of warts.

Warts and malignancy

Malignant change in warts is rare without immunosuppression. However, up to 90% of renal transplant patients develop warts within 5 years, and the sun then acts as a co-carcinogen. The association between anogenital warts and cervical neoplasia is mentioned below.

" Malignant change in warts is rare without immuno-suppression "

Prevention

Plantar warts should be covered by a plaster or a "verruca sock" before a communal shower or swimming pool is used. Shoes can be used in public places. Those with peri-ungual warts should not bite their nails or nail folds as this spreads the warts.

Treatment[1,2]

An ideal wart treatment would remove the wart without recurrence, leave no scar and induce life-long immunity.

However, evidence for the effectiveness of most commonly used local wart treatments is surprisingly weak. Most trials of cryotherapy, for example, have not compared it with other treatments, or with a placebo. The strongest evidence is that supporting the superiority of

" Those with peri-ungual warts should not bite their nails or nail folds as this spreads the warts "

115

simple topical treatments containing salicylic acid over placebo preparations. Salicylic acid is a keratolytic that slowly destroys infected epidermis, the subsequent irritation stimulating an immune response. Pooled data from six placebo controlled trials showed a cure rate of 71% with topical salicylic acid compared with 48% in the placebo treated controls.

One recent set of guidelines found the published evidence "inadequate to permit the development of clear rules for treating particular types of warts in specific sites in individuals of various ages," and clinical decisions have to be made without this assistance.

The following points are worth considering before treatment is started. Taken together, they make a fair case for leaving some warts untreated.

- Most warts clear spontaneously without leaving a scar, but this takes time. About 30% clear in 6 months, and 65% in 2 years.
- Treatment can be time-consuming, painful and leave scars.
- No treatment is 100% effective or right for all patients.
- Even with treatment, clearance requires an immune response: in the immunosuppressed some warts never go away.
- The least destructive treatments are the best on cosmetically important areas such as the face.

Some treatments used for common warts are described in Figures 97 to 100.

"Even with treatment, clearance requires an immune response"

Fig. 97. Points to consider when using salicylic acid to treat common warts.

Salicylic acid

- There is not enough evidence to compare the value of the many products on the market

- Paints should be applied once a day, after moistening for 5 minutes in hot water and removing dead tissue and old paint with an emery board

- Cover with a plaster on the soles but not elsewhere

Cryotherapy

- Always warn patients that cryotherapy hurts and can cause blisters

- Paring before cryotherapy increases the cure rate of plantar but not of other warts

- Use liquid nitrogen rather than CO_2 snow or a dimethyl ether/propane mixture

- Freezing is more effective in conjunction with a topical salicylic acid preparation

- Cotton buds and sprays are equally effective, but be careful with sprays near the eyes

- As the wart virus survives in liquid nitrogen, use a new swab for every dipping

- Freeze till a halo of frozen skin appears around the wart

- Two freeze/thaw cycles are more effective than one

- Treatment intervals should not be longer than 3 weeks

- Be careful when freezing peri-ungual warts as this can damage the nail matrix

Fig. 98. Points to consider when using cryotherapy to treat common warts.

Curettage and cautery

- Useful for filiform warts on the face and limbs, or for solitary, stubborn or painful warts elsewhere

- Use with extra care on the soles. Avoid leaving a painful scar on a weight-bearing area

- Surgical excision is never justified

Fig. 99. Points to consider when using curettage and cautery to treat common warts.

Fig. 100. Other, more specialist, therapies to treat common warts.

Other treatments best given by a specialist

- Intralesional bleomycin injection – may be justified for stubborn or painful warts, but it is painful

- Carbon dioxide or a pulsed dye laser

- Dinitrobenzene – a potent topical sensitizer

- 5-fluorouracil, intralesional interferon, and photodynamic therapy

Anogenital warts[3]

Most treatments will clear lesions within 1 to 6 months, but 20% to 30% of patients develop new ones or relapse thereafter. The remedies used most often now are those applied by the patients themselves: either podophyllotoxin (0.5% solution or 0.15% cream) or imiquimod (5% cream). Their clearance rates are similar, but imiquimod, which modifies the immune response, may have a lower relapse rate. However, it is also more expensive.

Cryotherapy, electro-surgery or laser treatment can be considered for stubborn cases. Patients should be screened for other sexually transmitted diseases, and use barrier protection with new sexual contacts. Despite an established association with cervical neoplasia, the presence of anogenital warts is not in itself an indication for more frequent cervical smear tests.

"Plantar warts: treatment should start with a preparation containing salicylic acid"

Plantar warts[4]

Treatment should start with a preparation containing salicylic acid, used by the patient at home for 2 or 3 months. Clearance rates are highest in fit young adults and in those whose warts are recent. Indications for more active treatments, such as cryotherapy, include pain, interference with function, embarrassment and failure to respond to salicylic acid. A useful way of dealing with multiple small plantar warts is to soak them for 10 minutes at night in a 4% formalin solution.

Plane warts

These are usually inconspicuous and can be left alone. Strong treatments can even spread them by the Köbner effect. Either a 2% to 5% salicylic acid cream or imiquimod cream may be worth trying for facial plane warts.

CASE STUDIES

Case study 1
Psoriasis

A 55-year-old woman comes to see her GP. She was diagnosed with psoriasis at age 14. This has flared intermittently, often associated with stressful life events. She has successfully used topical clobetasol propionate (Dermovate), betamethasone (Betnovate), dithranol and calcipotriol (Dovonex). Twenty years earlier she had a single course of UVB. Currently she uses daily emollients to a few areas of stable plaque psoriasis, and intermittent T-gel for her scalp.

66Currently she uses daily emollients to a few areas of stable plaque psoriasis, and intermittent T-gel for her scalp 99

News of her daughter's large wedding in 6 months had precipitated a flare and emotional distress. She is upset at losing control of her body, the ugliness of the lesions, how they make her feel and the reaction of other people. She comments that while waiting to be seen, she noticed that no-one sat near her. She felt the other patients were afraid of catching something from her. She is afraid of being "a monster" at her daughter's wedding and couldn't begin to think about the photographs.

She had a previous episode of depression in her 20s when she was trying to decide whether to have children, given the genetic predisposition of psoriasis, but has no overt symptoms of depression.

Examination

She was an anxious patient and obese with a BMI of 31. She had widespread erythematous plaques over her trunk and extensor surfaces of her arms and legs. Some of these had silver scales (see Figures 101 and 102). There were scales present in her scalp but no nail changes.

66 She was an anxious patient and obese with a BMI of 31 99

Management

Emotional support to help her through this difficult time was necessary. Her family were busy with the wedding preparations, so it was agreed that she should receive counselling at the practice and that she should contact the Psoriasis Association (see Appendix 3, page 157).

66Emotional support to help her through this difficult time was necessary 99

With the wedding still some time away PUVA or UVB would be excellent options in view of the widespread plaques. However, she felt unable to commit to visiting the hospital two or three times a week for light treatment.

Instead, she opted for intensive topical treatment. In the past she had found calcipotriol too irritating, so a change to talcalcitol (Curaderm) and a short course of once daily clobetasone butyrate (Eumovate) ointment was suggested.

An appointment was made with the community dermatology nurse to provide support and advice about topical products for the scalp and trunk and tertiary referral if these treatments were ineffective.

A dermatologist review could be arranged if UVB or PUVA treatment is agreed.

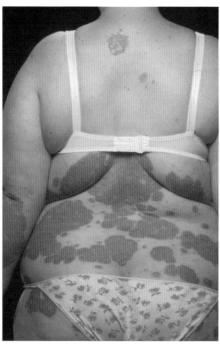

Fig. 101. Psoriasis over the back.

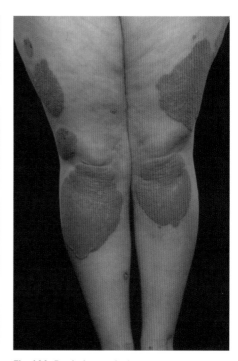

Fig. 102. Psoriasis over the legs.

Learning points

Psoriasis, like many chronic skin conditions, affects various aspects of a person's life. For example, many people suffer from low self-esteem. Support and education with input from the whole primary care team, and at times from the secondary care team, may help minimize the potential for disability.

Case study 2
Atypical mole syndrome and melanoma

A 24-year-old woman presents to her GP with a sports injury. As she is about to leave she mentions a mole that had become larger in the last few months. "I wouldn't bother you with it but my mother said I should mention it," she says.

She is otherwise fit and well and has no past medical history. Direct inquiry reveals she has multiple moles, but the one in question has enlarged and is itchy. Although not a sun-lover she previously worked as a postwoman. She had no significant family history, but reported that her father and brother also had multiple moles.

"Direct inquiry reveals she has multiple moles, but the one in question has enlarged and is itchy"

Examination

Her skin type was noted to be pale with freckles. She had multiple, large and unusually shaped moles over her trunk, consistent with atypical mole syndrome or dysplastic naevus syndrome (Figure 103). The mole that had changed was on her lower leg. It had an irregular outline, indistinct borders and measured 8.5mm (Figure 104). There were no palpable lymph nodes or hepatomegaly.

Management

The mole fulfilled the diagnostic criteria for a malignant melanoma (see Figure 56, page 68). She was referred to a dermatologist under the Government's 2-week urgent referral scheme, where immediate primary

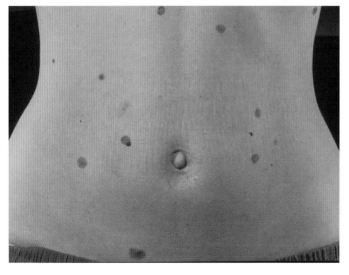

Fig. 103. Atypical mole syndrome seen on the patient's abdomen.

121

excision under local anaesthetic was performed on two of her moles. A full thickness excision biopsy was made with a 5mm margin of normal skin laterally. These were carefully labelled and sent for histology.

The patient was reviewed with the result of the biopsy. The mole of most concern was histologically a melanoma. The second biopsy was reported as a dysplastic naevus. The primary melanoma lesion had been completely excised. Breslow thickness was reported as 1.3mm (see Figure 57, page 68). She was referred for a further excision with 1.5cm margins. This was achieved without needing a skin graft.

Follow-up

"The 5-year survival rate for patients with a tumour of this type and depth lies between 80% and 96%"

The 5-year survival rate for patients with a tumour of this type and depth lies between 80% and 96%. Because she has atypical mole syndrome and a history of melanoma she has an increased risk of developing another melanoma. She had three monthly assessments at the pigmented lesion clinic for 3 years with 6-monthly photographs of her multiple moles to check for changes.

She was trained in mole self-examination. Her family was advised about the need for regular self-examination, and those with multiple moles were offered referral for monitoring by serial photography.

Fig. 104. Melanoma with an irregular outline and indistinct borders.

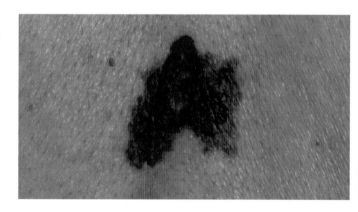

Learning points

Any mole that has changed must be carefully examined. A personal or family history of atypical mole syndrome or melanoma is important. Patients often place a low priority on skin conditions and are reluctant to present to their GP.

Case study 3
Lichen planus and NSAID use

A 55-year-old man presented with a 3-week history of itch and a rash. Initially, this was most noticeable around the ankles but more recently the right hand, especially around the wrist, was affected. The itch disrupted his sleep and did not settle with topical calamine lotion. There was no past or family history of skin problems. He was well and not on regular medications. No-one in his household had similar symptoms. He was unemployed and spent his days working on his allotment. There was no obvious flare in symptoms after gardening.

His GP initiated emollients and hydrocortisone 1% cream, which had no effect over 3 weeks. Re-attendance prompted treatment with Lyclear dermal cream and later an increase in topical steroid strength to clobetasone butyrate ointment (Eumovate).

When there was no improvement, he was referred to the dermatology clinic. On review there was little else to note, except that he had recently bought ibuprofen for a sore back. He had started taking this around the time the rash first presented. He hadn't thought to mention it when he was first asked about medications.

Examination
There were crops of raised papules around his ankles and wrist that had a lilac tint and a covering of fine white lines (Figure 105). There were also some scaly lesions, but no obvious scabies burrows. The oral mucosa had a white lace-like pattern (Figure 106) and the nails were unremarkable.

"The itch disrupted his sleep and did not settle with topical calamine lotion"

"When there was no improvement, he was referred to the dermatology clinic"

"Crops of raised papules around his ankles and wrist that had a lilac tint and a covering of fine white lines"

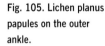

Fig. 105. Lichen planus papules on the outer ankle.

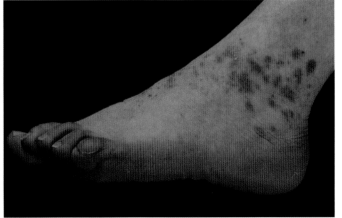

Fig. 106. Oral lesions of lichen planus.

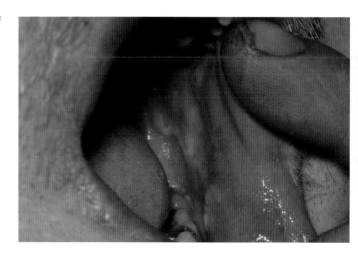

Management

Before the mouth was examined the diagnosis was likely to be lichen planus, but the differential diagnosis included psoriasis and nummular eczema. The oral lesions were diagnostic of lichen planus and this was confirmed with histology from a punch biopsy.

The potential exacerbating effect of the NSAID was discussed and the patient was happy to discontinue the drug and see his GP about alternative analgesia. He was aware that if he used this group of medication again, the skin condition could recur.

A sedating antihistamine was initiated to help alleviate the itch. Clobetasol propionate (Dermovate) ointment was applied twice daily. On review at 6 weeks the papules had flattened, and the itch was significantly reduced. The dose interval was therefore reduced to once weekly.

The patient was concerned about the dark pigmentation left where the lesions had been. It was explained that this would fade over the next few months. The oral lesions appeared to be less obvious and were likely to settle without specific treatment.

"A sedating antihistamine was initiated to help alleviate the itch"

"The patient was concerned about the dark pigmentation left where the lesions had been"

Learning points

This case illustrates the need to refer if the diagnosis is unclear or if first-line treatment does not improve symptoms. Potent topical steroids are usually needed to treat lichen planus. Drug eruption should be considered as a cause.

Case study 4

Contact dermatitis and tinea pedis

A 40-year-old man had suffered for some years from an intermittent rash under both feet. Usually it had started around the base of his big toes and then spread over both soles. It was extremely itchy, and burned especially when walking. In the past he had used OTC hydrocortisone cream with good effect, but this time the rash had become more extensive.

On examination, there was an erythematous scaly rash in a moccasin distribution (Figure 107), with no obvious vesicles, pustules or plaques.

Skin scrapings showed fungi on microscopy. For this reason the hydrocortisone cream was withdrawn and an imidazole cream was used instead. Later, as a subsequent report indicated that T. rubrum had been grown on culture, he took a 4-week course of terbinafine, 250mg daily. The rash improved, but did not clear fully and he was referred to a dermatologist.

Fungal scrapings were by now negative and the skin changes were felt to be eczematous. The possibility of an allergic contact dermatitis was considered in view of the long history of an intermittent rash responding to hydrocortisone. Patch testing was arranged: suspected antigens were applied to the patient's back under aluminium patches and left in place for 48 hours. The sites were inspected again at 96 hours and an assessment was made (Figure 108). This suggested a contact allergy to rubber. On direct questioning the patient said he had bought a new pair of slippers around the time the rash had flared most recently.

"Skin scrapings showed fungi on microscopy. For this reason the hydrocortisone cream was withdrawn and an imidazole cream was used instead"

"Patch testing suggested a contact allergy to rubber"

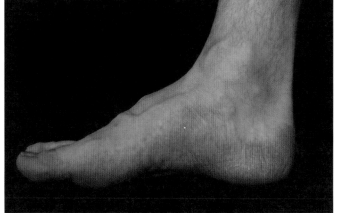

Fig. 107. Dermatitis on the foot in a moccasin-type distribution.

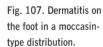

125

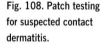

"Probably the use of a corticosteroid cream had allowed it to become so extensive"

Further management

The T. rubrum infection had by now been cleared. Probably the use of a corticosteroid cream had allowed it to become so extensive. An alternative, but perhaps less likely theory was that sensitization to rubber had been facilitated by the easier passage of allergens through skin already damaged by a fungal infection.

The patient was informed about contact allergy and a nurse explained how to apply the emollients and topical steroids required to treat his current rash. He was also advised not to use the slippers in question and to think carefully about every pair of shoes he owns. Sneakers and tennis shoes are obvious sources of rubber contact: less obvious ones are insoles and the rubber cements joining the shoe uppers, outer leather and lining. He will bear these facts in mind when he buys new shoes in the future, and will check carefully for a rash over the first few days of wearing them. He was asked to dispose of the socks he had worn with the shoes containing rubber, as washing does not always remove rubber particles completely.

He was also given general advice about other rubber products, as he will be at risk when any part of his body comes into contact with them. Finally, as he worked as a healthcare assistant, he was concerned about latex allergy. He was reassured about this.

Fig. 108. Patch testing for suspected contact dermatitis.

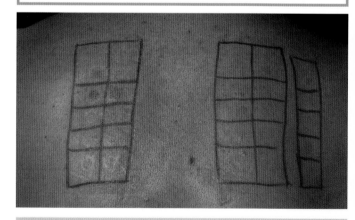

Learning points

Contact allergies can be difficult to differentiate from other skin disorders. Skin infections can confuse the issue further. Patch testing is a useful investigation for Type IV delayed hypersensitivity reactions, but requires a specialist to interpret the results accurately.

DRUG TABLES

Emollients and soap substitutes

Emollients are best applied after a bath or shower and should be used liberally. They help those with dry and itchy skin conditions. Some can be used as soap substitutes.

Emollients and soap substitutes

Emollient	Can be used as a soap substitute	Comments
Dermol 500 lotion, Dermol 200 shower emollient	Dermol 500 lotion, Dermol 200 shower emollient	Contain benzalkonium and chlorhexidine. For use, therefore, when infection is likely
Aqueous cream, emulsifying ointment, hydrous ointment (oily cream), liquid/white soft paraffin, white soft paraffin, yellow soft paraffin ointment	Aqueous cream, emulsifying ointment	Generic preparations
Aveeno cream and lotion (contain oatmeal), Cetraban cream, Dermamist spray, Diprobase cream, Doublebase gel, E45 lotion and cream, Epaderm ointment, Hydromol cream, Keri lotion, Lipobase cream, Oilatum cream, Unguentum M cream, Ultrabase cream	E45 Skin Wash Cream, Epaderm ointment, Oilatum shower gel	Proprietary preparations
Aquadrate cream, Balneum Plus cream, Calmurid cream, E45 Itch Relief cream. Eucerin cream and lotion		Contain urea, a hydrating agent used in scaly conditions

Emollient bath additives

Emollient bath additive	Comments
Alpha Keri bath oil, Aveeno bath oil (contains oatmeal), Balneum bath oil, Balneum Plus bath oil, Diprobath bath additive, E45 emollient bath oil, Hydromol Emollient bath additive, Oilatum Emollient bath additive	Proprietary preparations
Dermol 600 bath emollient, Emulsiderm liquid emulsion, Oilatum plus bath additive	Contain benzalkonium. For use, therefore, when infection is likely

Topical corticosteroids

Drug	Trade name	Preparation	Strength	Conditions and doses	Comments	Side-effects
Aclometasone dipropionate	Modrasone	Cream	0.05%	Inflammatory skin conditions: apply sparingly 1–2 times/d	Moderate potency; contraindicated in untreated bacterial, fungal or viral skin lesions, acne rosacea, perioral dermatitis, acne vulgaris; caution in prolonged use and use on face	See hydrocortisone
		Ointment	0.05%			
Betamethasone dipropionate	Diprosone	Cream	0.05%	Severe inflammatory skin conditions such as eczemas unresponsive to less potent corticosteroids, psoriasis: apply sparingly 1–2 times/d	Potent; contraindicated in untreated bacterial, fungal or viral skin lesions, acne rosacea, perioral dermatitis, acne vulgaris; caution in prolonged use and use on face	See hydrocortisone; application of >200g/week of a 0.05% preparation (or equivalent) likely to cause adrenal suppression
		Ointment	0.05%			
		Lotion	0.05%			
Betamethasone dipropionate and salicylic acid	Diprosalic	Cream	0.05% + 3%	As above: apply sparingly 1–2 times/d (max 60g/week)	Salicylic acid increases the corticosteroid penetration	
		Lotion	0.05% + 2%	As above: apply a few drops 1–2 times/d		
Betamethasone dipropionate and clotrimazole	Lotriderm	Cream	0.064% + 1%	Severe inflammatory conditions with associated fungal infection: apply sparingly 1–2 times/d		

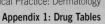

Drug	Trade name	Preparation	Strength	Conditions and doses	Comments	Side-effects
Betamethasone valerate	Generic	Cream	0.1%	Severe inflammatory skin conditions such as eczemas unresponsive to less potent corticosteroids; psoriasis: apply sparingly 1–2 times/d	Potent; contraindicated in untreated bacterial, fungal or viral skin lesions, acne rosacea, perioral dermatitis, acne vulgaris; caution in prolonged use and use on face	See hydrocortisone; application of >100g/week of a 0.1% preparation likely to cause adrenal suppression
		Ointment	0.1%			
	Betacap	Scalp application	0.1%			
	Betnovate	Cream	0.1%			
		Ointment	0.1%			
		Lotion	0.1%			
		Scalp application	0.1%			
	Betnovate RD	Cream	0.025%	Inflammatory skin disorders: apply sparingly 1–2 times/d	Moderate potency	
		Ointment	0.025%			
	Betta-mousse	Scalp application	0.1%		Potent	
	Betnovate C	Cream	0.1% + 0.5%	Severe inflammatory conditions with associated infection: apply sparingly 1–2 times/d	Potent	
		Ointment	0.1% + 0.5%			
Betamethasone valerate + clioquinol	Betnovate N	Cream	0.1% + 0.5%	Severe inflammatory conditions with associated infection: apply sparingly 1–2 times/d	Potent	
		Ointment	0.1% + 0.5%			
Betamethasone valerate + neomycin	Fucibet	Cream	0.1% + 0.5%	Severe inflammatory conditions with associated infection: apply sparingly 1–2 times/d	Potent	
Betamethasone + fusidic acid						

129

Drug	Trade name	Preparation	Strength	Conditions and doses	Comments	Side-effects
Clobetasol propionate	Dermovate	Cream	0.05%	Short-term treatment of severe resistant inflammatory skin disorders such as recalcitrant eczemas unresponsive to less potent corticosteroids;	Very potent; contra-indicated in untreated bacterial, fungal or viral skin lesions, acne rosacea, perioral dermatitis, acne vulgaris; caution in prolonged use and use on face	See hydrocortisone
		Ointment	0.05%			
		Scalp application	0.05%	psoriasis: apply sparingly 1–2 times/d for up to 4 weeks (max 50g of 0.05% preparation/week)		
Clobetasol propionate + neomycin + nystatin	Dermovate NN	Cream	0.05% + 0.05% + 100000u/g	Short-term treatment of severe resistant inflammatory conditions with associated infection: apply sparingly 1–2 times/d		
		Ointment	0.05% + 0.05% + 100000u/g			
Clobetasone butyrate	Eumovate	Cream	0.05%	Eczemas and dermatitis of all types; maintenance between courses of more potent corticosteroids: apply sparingly 1–2 times/d	Moderate potency; contraindicated in untreated bacterial, fungal or viral skin lesions, acne rosacea, perioral dermatitis, acne vulgaris; caution in prolonged use and use on face	See hydrocortisone
		Ointment	0.05%			
Clobetasone butyrate + oxytetracycline + nystatin	Trimovate	Cream	0.05% + 3% + 100000u/g	Severe inflammatory conditions with associated infection: apply sparingly 1–2 times/d		Stains clothing
Desoximetasone	Stiedex LP	Oily cream	0.05%	Severe acute inflammatory, allergic and chronic skin disorders; psoriasis: apply sparingly 1–2 times/d	Potent; contraindicated in untreated bacterial, fungal or viral skin lesions, acne rosacea, perioral dermatitis, acne vulgaris; caution in prolonged use and use on face; salicylic acid increases corticosteroid penetration	See hydrocortisone
Desoximetasone + salicylic acid	Stiedex	Lotion	0.25% + 1%			

Drug	Trade name	Preparation	Strength	Conditions and doses	Comments	Side-effects
Diflucortolone valerate	Nerisone	Cream	0.1%	Severe inflammatory skin disorders such as eczemas unresponsive to less potent corticosteroids; apply sparingly 1–2 times/d for up to 4 weeks	Potent (0.1%), very potent (0.3%); contraindicated in untreated bacterial, fungal or viral skin lesions, acne rosacea, perioral dermatitis, acne vulgaris; caution in prolonged use and use on face	See hydrocortisone
		Oily cream	0.1%			
		Ointment	0.1%			
	Nerisone Forte	Oily cream	0.3%	Short term treatment of severe exacerbations of inflammatory skin disorders; apply sparingly 1–2 times/d for up to 2 weeks (max 60g/week)		
		Ointment	0.3%			
Fludroxycortide (flurandrenolone)	Haelan	Cream	0.0125%	Inflammatory skin disorders: apply sparingly 1–2 times/d	Moderate potency; contraindicated in untreated bacterial, fungal or viral skin lesions, acne rosacea, perioral dermatitis, acne vulgaris; caution in prolonged use and use on face	See hydrocortisone
		Ointment	0.0125%			

Drug	Trade name	Preparation	Strength	Conditions and doses	Comments	Side-effects
Fluocinolone acetonide	Synalar	Cream	0.025%	Inflammatory skin disorders; psoriasis: apply sparingly 1–2 times/d, reduce strength as condition responds	Potent (0.025%), moderate potency (0.00625%), mild (0.0025%); contraindicated in untreated bacterial, fungal or viral skin lesions, acne rosacea, perioral dermatitis, acne vulgaris; caution in prolonged use and use on face	See hydrocortisone
		Gel	0.025%			
		Ointment	0.025%			
	Synalar 1 in 4 Dilution	Cream	0.00625%			
	Synalar 1 in 10 Dilution	Cream	0.0025%			
Fluocinolone acetate + clioquinol	Synalar C	Cream	0.025% + 3%	Inflammatory conditions with associated infection: apply sparingly 1–2 times/d		
		Ointment	0.025% + 3%			
Fluocinolone acetate + neomycin	Synalar N	Cream	0.025% + 0.5%			
		Ointment	0.025% + 0.5%			
Fluticasone propionate	Cutivate	Cream	0.05%	Inflammatory skin disorders such as dermatitis and eczemas unresponsive to less potent corticosteroids: apply cream sparingly once daily or ointment 2 times/d	Potent; contraindicated in untreated bacterial, fungal or viral skin lesions, acne rosacea, perioral dermatitis, acne vulgaris; caution in prolonged use and use on face	See hydrocortisone
		Ointment	0.005%			

Drug	Trade name	Preparation	Strength	Conditions and doses	Comments	Side-effects
Hydrocortisone	Generic	Cream	0.5%, 1%	Mild inflammatory skin disorders such as eczemas: apply sparingly 1-2 times/d	Mild; contraindicated in untreated bacterial, fungal or viral skin lesions, acne rosacea, perioral dermatitis, acne vulgaris; caution in prolonged use and use on face	Systemic absorption and skin thinning following prolonged use, worsening of untreated infection
		Ointment	0.5%, 1%			
	Dioderm	Cream	0.1% (equivalent to 1% due to formulation)			
	Efcortelan	Cream	0.5%, 1%, 2.5%			
		Ointment	0.5%, 1%, 2.5%			
Hydrocortisone + clotrimazole	Canesten HC	Cream	1% + 1%	Mild inflammatory skin disorders with associated fungal infection		
Hydrocortisone + crotamiton	Eurax HC	Cream	0.25% + 10%	Mild inflammatory skin disorders with itching		
Hydrocortisone + econazole	Econacort	Cream	1% + 1%	Mild inflammatory skin disorders with associated fungal infection		
Hydrocortisone + fusidic acid	Fucidin H	Cream	1% + 2%	Mild inflammatory skin disorders with associated bacterial infection		
		Ointment	1% + 2%			
Hydrocortisone + miconazole	Daktacort	Cream	1% + 2%	Mild inflammatory skin disorders with associated fungal infection		
		Ointment	1% + 2%			
Hydrocortisone + nystatin	Timodine	Cream	0.5% + 100000u/g	Mild inflammatory skin disorders with associated fungal infection		
Hydrocortisone + urea	Alphaderm	Cream	1% + 10%	Mild inflammatory skin disorders with itching		
Hydrocortisone + urea	Calmurid HC	Cream	1% + 10%	Mild inflammatory skin disorders with itching		

Drug	Trade name	Preparation	Strength	Conditions and doses	Comments	Side-effects
Hydrocortisone butyrate	Locoid	Cream	0.1%	Mild inflammatory skin disorders such as eczemas: apply sparingly 1–2 times/d	Mild; contraindicated in untreated bacterial, fungal or viral skin lesions, acne rosacea, perioral dermatitis, acne vulgaris; caution in prolonged use and use on face	See hydrocortisone
		Lipocream	0.1%			
		Ointment	0.1%			
		Scalp lotion	0.1%			
Hydrocortisone butyrate + clioquinol	Locoid C	Cream	0.1% + 3%	Mild inflammatory skin disorders with associated infection		Causes staining
		Ointment	0.1% + 3%			
Mometasone furoate	Elocon	Cream	0.1%	Severe inflammatory skin disorders such as eczemas unresponsive to less potent corticosteroids; psoriasis: apply sparingly once daily	Potent; contraindicated in untreated bacterial, fungal or viral skin lesions, acne rosacea, perioral dermatitis, acne vulgaris; caution in prolonged use and use on face	See hydrocortisone
		Ointment	0.1%			
		Scalp lotion	0.1%			

Other preparations for eczema

Drug	Trade name	Preparation	Strength	Conditions and doses	Comments	Side-effects
Doxepin	Xepin	Cream	5%	Pruritus in eczema: apply sparingly 3–4 times/d (max 3g/application; total max 12g/d; coverage should be <10% of body surface area)	Caution in glaucoma, urinary retention, severe hepatic impairment, pregnancy and breast feeding	Drowsiness, local burning, stinging, irritation, rash; dry mouth and other systemic side-effects
Ichthammol	Generic	Cream	5%	Chronic lichenified eczema: apply 1–2 times/d		Skin irritation
		Ointment	10%			

Drug	Trade name	Preparation	Strength	Conditions and doses	Comments	Side-effects
Pimecrolimus	Elidel	Cream	1%	Mild to moderate atopic eczema and to prevent flares: apply 2 times/d until symptoms resolve (not a first-line treatment)	Contraindicated if treatment site is infected, congenital epidermal barrier defects, generalized erythroderma; avoid contact with eyes and mucous membranes, avoid excessive exposure to UV light, do not apply under occlusion	Burning sensation, pruritus, erythema, skin infections, local reactions (pain, paraesthesia, peeling, dryness, oedema and worsening of eczema)
Tacrolimus	Protopic	Ointment	0.03%, 0.1%	Moderate to severe atopic eczema: apply 0.1% preparation sparingly 2 times/d for up to 3 weeks then use the 0.03% preparation 1–2 times/d until lesions clear (not a first-line treatment)	Contraindicated if treatment site is infected, congenital epidermal barrier defects, generalized erythroderma, pregnancy and breast feeding; avoid contact with eyes and mucous membranes, avoid excessive exposure to UV light, do not apply under occlusion	Burning and tingling sensations, pruritus, erythema, folliculitis, acne, predisposition to herpes simplex infections, increased sensitivity to hot and cold, alcohol intolerance, lymphadenopathy

Topical preparations for psoriasis

Drug	Trade name	Preparation	Strength	Conditions and doses	Comments	Side-effects
Calcipotriol	Dovonex	Cream	50mcg/g	Mild to moderate plaque psoriasis: apply 1–2 times/d to max 35% of body surface (max 30g/d or calcipotriol 5mg when used with scalp application)	Contraindicated in disorders of calcium metabolism; do not use on face or under occlusion; caution in pregnancy, hepatic and renal impairment	Local irritation, dermatitis, pruritus, erythema, burning, paraesthesia, aggravation of psoriasis, photosensitivity, facial or perioral dermatitis, hyperkalaemia
		Ointment	50mcg/g			
		Scalp application	50mcg/g	Mild to moderate plaque psoriasis; apply 2 times/d (max 60ml/week)		
	Silkis	Ointment	3mcg/g			
Calcipotriol + betamethasone	Dovobet	Ointment	50mcg/g + 0.05%	Initial treatment of stable plaque psoriasis: apply once daily to max 30% of body surface (max 15g/d) for up to 4 weeks	See above and under betamethasone	See above and under betamethasone
Coal tar	Alphosyl	Cream	5% (+ allantoin)	Apply 2–4 times/d	Contraindicated on sore, acute or pustular psoriasis or in presence of infection; caution to avoid eyes, mucosa, genital and rectal areas and broken or inflamed skin	Skin irritation and acne-like eruptions, photosensitivity, stains skin, hair and fabric
		Lotion	5% (+ allantoin)			
	Carbo-Dome	Cream	10%	Apply 2–3 times/d		
	Clinitar	Cream	1%	Apply 1–2 times/d		
	Cocois	Scalp application	12% (+ salicylic acid and sulphur)	Scaly scalp disorders including psoriasis, eczema, seborrhoeic dermatitis and dandruff: apply once weekly		
	Exorex	Lotion	1%	Apply 2–3 times/d		
	Polytar Emollient	Bath additive	7.5% (+ arachis oil, cade oil and liquid paraffin)	Psoriasis, eczema, atopic and pruritic dermatoses: add 15–30ml to bath and soak for 20min		

Drug	Trade name	Preparation	Strength	Conditions and doses	Comments	Side-effects
Dithranol	Dithro-cream	Cream	0.1%, 0.25%, 0.5%, 1%, 2%	Apply to skin or scalp; 0.1–0.5% preparations can be left on overnight and 1–2% left on for max 1h; start treatment with low strengths	Contraindicated in acute and pustular psoriasis; caution to avoid eyes and sensitive areas of skin	Local burning sensation and irritation, stains skin, hair and fabrics
Tacalcitol	Curatoderm	Ointment	4mcg/g	Plaque psoriasis: apply once daily (max 10g/d)	Contraindicated in disorders of calcium metabolism; do not use on face or under occlusion; caution in pregnancy, hepatic and renal impairment	Local irritation, dermatitis, pruritus, erythema, burning, paraesthesia, aggravation of psoriasis, photosensitivity, facial or perioral dermatitis, hyperkalaemia
Tazarotene	Zorac	Gel	0.05%, 0.1%	Mild to moderate psoriasis affecting <10% of body surface: apply once daily for up to 12 weeks	Contraindicated in pregnancy and breast feeding; caution to avoid eyes, face, eczematous or inflamed skin; do not apply within an hour of using emollients	**Teratogenic** — women of childbearing age should use contraceptive protection; local irritation, pruritus, burning, erythema, desquamation, non-specific rash, contact dermatitis, worsening of psoriasis, stinging, skin inflammation

Oral treatments for psoriasis

Drug	Trade name	Preparation	Strength	Conditions and doses	Comments	Side-effects
Acitretin	Neotigason	Capsule	10mg, 25mg	**Under expert supervision:** severe extensive psoriasis resistant to other forms of therapy; palmoplantar pustular psoriasis; pustular psoriasis; severe congenital ichthyosis: 25–30mg/d for 2–4 weeks then adjust according to response (usual range 25–50mg/d, max 75mg/d) for further 6–8 weeks	Contraindicated in pregnancy and breast feeding, hepatic and renal impairment, hyperlipidaemia	**Teratogenic** — women of childbearing age should use contraception for at least 1 month before treatment, during treatment and for 2 years after completing treatment; hepatic dysfunction (monitor lipids), dryness of mucous membranes, skin erosion, erythema, conjunctivitis
Ciclosporin	Neoral	Capsule	10mg, 25mg, 50mg, 100mg	**Under expert supervision:** short-term treatment severe atopic dermatitis when conventional therapy is ineffective: 2.5mg/kg/d (max 5mg/kg/d for max 8 weeks); severe psoriasis when conventional therapy is ineffective: 2.5mg/kg/d (max 5mg/kg/d)	Contraindicated in uncontrolled hypertension, uncontrolled infections and malignancy, renal impairment, allow skin infections to clear before starting treatment	Increased serum creatinine and urea (monitor renal function), hypertrichosis, tremor, hypertension, hepatic dysfunction, fatigue, gingival hypertrophy, gastrointestinal disturbances
Methotrexate	Maxtrex	Tablet	2.5mg, 10mg	**Specialist use only:** severe uncontrolled psoriasis unresponsive to conventional therapy: 10–25mg once **weekly** and adjusted according to response	Contraindicated in pregnancy and breast feeding, active infection and immunodeficiency syndromes; caution in blood disorders, renal disorders, peptic ulceration, ulcerative colitis	**Teratogenic** — men and women of childbearing potential should avoid conception for at least 3 months after completing treatment; blood dyscrasias (monitor blood count), liver cirrhosis (monitor hepatic function), pulmonary toxicity

Topical preparations for acne

Drug	Trade name	Preparation	Strength	Conditions and doses	Comments	Side-effects
Adapalene	Differin	Cream	0.1%	Mild to moderate acne: apply sparingly at night	Contraindicated in pregnancy, cutaneous epithelioma, in severe, widespread acne; caution to avoid contact with eyes, mouth and mucous membranes, avoid UV light	Local reactions (burning, erythema, stinging, pruritus, dry or peeling skin, increased sensitivity to UV light, temporary changes in skin pigmentation)
		Gel	0.1%			
Azelaic acid	Skinoren	Cream	20%	Acne vulgaris: apply 2 times/d for max 6 months	Caution in pregnancy and breast feeding	Local irritation
Benzoyl peroxide	Brevoxyl	Cream	4%	Acne vulgaris: apply 1–2 times/d after washing with soap and water; start treatment with lower strength preparations	Caution to avoid contact with eyes, mouth and mucous membranes, may bleach hair and fabrics, avoid excessive exposure to sunlight	Skin irritation; most preparations contain excipients that rarely cause skin sensitisation
	PanOxyl	Aquagel	2.5%, 5%, 10%			
		Cream	5%, 10%			
		Gel	5%, 10%			
		Wash	10%			
Clindamycin	Dalacin T	Solution	1%	Apply 2 times/d		Mild skin irritation, skin sensitisation
		Lotion	1%			
Erythromycin	Stiemycin	Solution	2%	Apply 2 times/d		Mild skin irritation, skin sensitisation
	Zineryt	Solution	1.3%	Apply 2 times/d		

Drug	Trade name	Preparation	Strength	Conditions and doses	Comments	Side-effects
Isotretinoin	Isotrex	Gel	0.05%	Mild to moderate acne: apply sparingly 1–2 times/d	Contraindicated in pregnancy, cutaneous epithelioma, in severe, widespread acne; caution to avoid contact with eyes, mouth and mucous membranes, avoid UV light	**Teratogenic** — women of childbearing age should take adequate contraceptive measures; local reactions (burning, erythema, stinging, pruritus, dry or peeling skin, increased sensitivity to UV light, temporary changes in skin pigmentation)
Isotretinoin + erythromycin	Isotrexin	Gel	0.05% + 2%			
	Aknemycin Plus	Lotion	0.025% + 4%			
Nicotinamide	Nicam	Gel	4%	Inflammatory acne vulgaris: apply 2 times/d reducing to once daily if irritation occurs	Caution to avoid contact with eyes and mucous membranes	Dry skin, erythema, pruritus, burning, irritation
Tetracycline	Topicycline	Solution	2.2%	Apply 2 times/d		Mild skin irritation, skin sensitisation
Tretinoin	Retin-A	Cream	0.025%	Acne vulgaris and other keratotic conditions: apply sparingly 1–2 times/d (use lower strengths for dry or fair skin)	Contraindicated in pregnancy, cutaneous epithelioma, in severe, widespread acne; caution to avoid contact with eyes, mouth and mucous membranes, avoid UV light	**Teratogenic** — women of childbearing age should take adequate contraceptive measures; local reactions (burning, erythema, stinging, pruritus, dry or peeling skin, increased sensitivity to UV light, temporary changes in skin pigmentation)
		Gel	0.01%, 0.02%			
		Lotion	0.025%			
	Retinova	Cream	0.05%	Photo-damaged skin: apply sparingly at night, reducing to 1–3 nights weekly		

Oral preparations for acne

Drug	Trade name	Preparation	Strength	Conditions and doses	Comments	Side-effects
Cyproterone + ethinylestradiol (co-cyprindiol)	Dianette	Tablet	2mg + 35mcg	Severe acne in women refractory to prolonged antibacterial therapy: I tablet/d for 21 days and repeat after a 7-day interval	Contraindications and cautions of combined oral contraceptives; women with severe acne may have an inherently increased risk of cardiovascular disease	Side-effects of oral contraceptives
Doxycycline	Vibramycin	Capsule	50mg, 100mg	Inflammatory acne: 100mg/d	Contraindicated in pregnancy and breast feeding, renal impairment; caution in hepatic impairment	Nausea, vomiting, diarrhoea, dysphagia, oesophageal irritation, hypersensitivity reactions, hepatotoxicity, photosensitivity
Erythromycin	Generic	Tablet	250mg	Acne and rosacea: 500mg 2 times/d	Caution in renal and hepatic impairment, pregnancy and breast feeding	Nausea, vomiting, abdominal discomfort, diarrhoea, urticaria, rashes and other allergic reactions
	Erymax	Capsule	250mg			
Isotretinoin	Roaccutane	Capsule	5mg, 20mg	**Under expert supervision:** Nodulo-cystic and conglobate acne, severe acne, scarring, acne that has not responded to systemic antimicrobial therapy and acne that is associated with psychological problems: 0.5mg/kg/d for 4 weeks increasing to max 1mg/kg/d for 8–12 weeks	Contraindicated in pregnancy, breast feeding, hepatic and renal impairment, hypervitaminosis, hyperlipidaemia; caution in diabetes, dry eye syndrome, avoid keratolytics	**Teratogenic** — women of childbearing age should use contraception for at least 1 month before treatment, during treatment and for 1 month after completing treatment; hepatic dysfunction (monitor lipids), dryness of skin, epithelial fragility, conjunctivitis, nausea, neadache, malaise, drowsiness

Drug	Trade name	Preparation	Strength	Conditions and doses	Comments	Side-effects
Minocycline	Generic	Tablet	50mg, 100mg	Acne: 100mg/d	Contraindicated in pregnancy and breast feeding, caution in hepatic impairment	Nausea, vomiting, diarrhoea, dysphagia, oesophageal irritation, hypersensitivity reactions, hepatotoxicity, skin pigmentation, discolouration of conjunctiva
	Aknemin	Capsule	50mg			
	Minocin MR	M/R capsule	100mg			
Oxytetracycline	Generic	Tablet	250mg	Acne: 500mg 2 times/d	Contraindicated in pregnancy and breast feeding, renal impairment; caution in hepatic impairment	Nausea, vomiting, diarrhoea, dysphagia, oesophageal irritation, hypersensitivity reactions, hepatotoxicity
Tetracycline	Generic	Tablet	250mg	Acne: 250mg 2 times/d	Contraindicated in pregnancy and breast feeding, renal impairment; caution in hepatic impairment	Nausea, vomiting, diarrhoea, dysphagia, oesophageal irritation, hypersensitivity reactions, hepatotoxicity

Preparations for warts and calluses

Drug	Trade name	Preparation	Strength	Conditions and doses	Comments	Side-effects
Formaldehyde	Veracur	Gel	0.75%	Plantar warts: apply 2 times/d		Skin irritation
Glutaraldehyde	Glutarol	Solution	10%	Plantar warts: apply 2 times/d		Skin irritation, stains skin brown

Drug	Trade name	Preparation	Strength	Conditions and doses	Comments	Side-effects
Salicylic acid	Cuplex	Gel	11% (+ lactic acid 4%)	Plantar and mosaic warts, corns and calluses: apply 2 times/d	Contraindicated in diabetes and impaired peripheral blood circulation; caution to avoid broken skin and protect surrounding areas	Skin irritation
	Duofilm	Paint	16.7% (+ lactic acid 16.7%)	Plantar and mosaic warts: apply daily		
	Occlusal	Application	26%	Plantar warts: apply daily		
	Salactol	Paint	16.7% (+ lactic acid 16.7%)	Plantar warts, verrucas, corns and calluses: apply daily		
	Salatac	Gel	12% (+ lactic acid 4%)	Warts, verrucas, corns and calluses: apply daily		
	Verrugon	Ointment	50%	Plantar warts: apply daily		
Silver nitrate	AVOCA	Caustic pencil	95%	Apply moistened caustic pencil tip for 1–2min repeat after 24h up to max 3 applications (warts) or 6 applications (verrucas)	Protect surrounding skin and avoid broken skin	Stains skin and fabric

Preparations for photodamaged skin

Drug	Trade name	Preparation	Strength	Conditions and doses	Comments	Side-effects
Diclofenac	Solaraze	Gel	3%	Actinic keratosis: apply sparingly 2 times/d for 60–90 days (max 8g/d)	Caution in asthma; avoid contact with eyes, mucous membranes and inflamed skin	Hypersensitivity reactions, paraesthesia
Fluorouracil	Efudix	Cream	5%	Actinic keratosis: apply sparingly 1–2 times/d (max area of skin treated 500 cm2)		Local irritation, mucositis

Drug	Trade name	Preparation	Strength	Conditions and doses	Comments	Side-effects
Tretinoin	Retinova	Cream	0.05%	Apply sparingly at night, reducing to 1–3 nights weekly	Contraindicated in pregnancy, cutaneous epithelioma, in severe, widespread acne; caution to avoid contact with eyes, mouth and mucous membranes, avoid UV light	**Teratogenic** — women of childbearing age should take adequate contraceptive measures; local reactions (burning, erythema, stinging, pruritus, dry or peeling skin, increased sensitivity to UV light, temporary changes in skin pigmentation)

Alopecia

Drug	Trade name	Preparation	Strength	Conditions and doses	Comments	Side-effects
Finasteride	Propecia	Tablet	1mg	Male pattern baldness: 1mg/d for 3–6 months	For use in men only; caution in obstructive uropathy and prostate cancer; effects reversed 6–12 months after stopping treatment	Impotence, decreased libido, ejaculation disorders, testicular pain, breast tenderness and enlargement, hypersensitivity reactions
Minoxidil	Regaine	Topical Solution		Male pattern baldness in men and women (2% only): apply 1ml 2 times/d to dry hair and scalp	Caution to avoid contact with eyes, mouth and mucous membranes, broken infected or inflamed skin	Irritant dermatitis, allergic contact dermatitis, discontinue if hair loss persists for >2 weeks

Topical antibacterial preparations

Drug	Trade name	Preparation	Strength	Conditions and doses	Comments	Side-effects
Fusidic acid	Fucidin	Cream	2%	Bacterial skin infections (e.g. impetigo): apply 3–4 times/d	Caution to avoid contact with eyes; may be used with oral antibiotics (e.g. flucloxacillin) for deeper infections	Skin irritation
		Gel	2%			
		Ointment	2%			
Metronidazole	Anabact	Gel	0.75%	Malodorous fungating tumours and ulcers: apply 1–2 times daily and cover with non-adherent dressing	Caution to avoid exposure to strong sunlight or UV light	
	Metrogel	Gel	0.75%	Acute inflammatory exacerbations of acne rosacea: apply sparingly daily for 8–9 weeks		
	Metrosa	Gel	0.75%	Acute inflammatory exacerbations of acne rosacea: apply sparingly 2 times/d for 8–9 weeks		
	Metrotop	Gel	0.8%	Malodorous fungating tumours and ulcers: apply 1–2 times daily and cover with non-adherent dressing		
	Noritate	Cream	1%	Acne rosacea: apply daily for 8 weeks		
	Rozex	Cream	0.75%	Inflammatory papules, pustules and erythema of acne rosacea: apply 2 times/d for 3–4 months		
		Gel	0.75%			
Mupirocin	Bactroban	Cream	2%	Bacterial skin infections (e.g. impetigo and secondarily infected traumatic lesions): apply 2–3 times/d for max 10 days	May be used with oral antibiotics (e.g. flucloxacillin) for deeper infections	
		Ointment	2%			

Topical antifungal preparations

Drug	Trade name	Preparation	Strength	Conditions and doses	Comments	Side-effects
Clotrimazole	Canesten	Cream	1%	Fungal skin infections (e.g. candidiasis, dermatophytoses and pityriasis versicolor): apply 2–3 times/d	Caution to avoid contact with eyes and mucous membranes; may be used with systemic antifungals for deeper infections	Local irritation and hypersensitivity reactions (mild burning, erythema, itching)
		Powder	1%			
		Solution	1%			
Econazole	Ecostatin	Cream	1%	Fungal skin infections (e.g. candidiasis, dermatophytoses and pityriasis versicolor): apply 2 times/d	Caution to avoid contact with eyes and mucous membranes; may be used with systemic antifungals for deeper infections	Local irritation and hypersensitivity reactions (mild burning, erythema, itching)
	Pevaryl	Cream	1%			
Ketoconazole	Nizoral	Cream	2%	Fungal skin infections (e.g. candidiasis, dermatophytoses and pityriasis versicolor): apply 1–2 times/d	Caution to avoid contact with eyes and mucous membranes; may be used with systemic antifungals for deeper infections	Local irritation and hypersensitivity reactions (mild burning, erythema, itching)
Miconazole	Daktarin	Cream	2%	Fungal skin infections (e.g. candidiasis, dermatophytoses and pityriasis versicolor): apply 2 times/d continuing for 10 days after lesions have healed	Caution to avoid contact with eyes and mucous membranes; may be used with systemic antifungals for deeper infections	Local irritation and hypersensitivity reactions (mild burning, erythema, itching)
		Powder	2%			
Nystatin	Nystan	Cream	100000u/g	Candidiasis: apply 2–4 times/d	Caution to avoid contact with eyes and mucous membranes; may be used with systemic antifungals for deeper infections	Local irritation and ersensitivity reactions (mild burning, erythema, itching)
		Ointment	100000u/g			

Drug	Trade name	Preparation	Strength	Conditions and doses	Comments	Side-effects
Sulconazole	Exelderm	Cream	1%	Fungal skin infections (e.g. candidiasis, dermatophytoses and pityriasis versicolor): apply 1–2 times/d continuing for 2–3 weeks after lesions have healed	Caution to avoid contact with eyes and mucous membranes; may be used with systemic antifungals for deeper infections	Local irritation and hypersensitivity reactions (mild burning, erythema, itching), blistering
Terbinafine	Lamisil	Cream	1%	Fungal skin infections (e.g. candidiasis, dermatophytoses and pityriasis versicolor): apply 1–2 times/d for up to 2 weeks	Caution in pregnancy and breast feeding, avoid contact with eyes; may be used with systemic antifungals for deeper infections	Local irritation and hypersensitivity reactions (erythema, itching, stinging)

Oral antifungal preparations

Drug	Trade name	Preparation	Strength	Conditions and doses	Comments	Side-effects
Fluconazole	Generic	Capsule	50mg, 150mg, 200mg	Tinea pedis, corporis, cruris, pityriasis versicolor, dermal candidiasis: 50mg/d for 2–4 weeks (max 6 weeks)	Caution in hepatic and renal impairment, pregnancy, breast feeding, monitor liver function	Nausea, abdominal discomfort, diarrhoea, flatulence, rash
	Diflucan	Capsule	50mg, 150mg, 200mg			
Griseofulvin	Grisovin	Tablet	125mg, 500mg	Dermatophyte infections of skin, scalp, hair, nails: 500mg/d (double in severe infections and reduce when response occurs)	Contraindicated in severe liver disease, lupus erythematosus, porphyria, pregnancy; caution in breast feeding	**Teratogenic:** avoid during and for 1 month after pregnancy, men should not father children within 6 months of treatment; headache, nausea, vomiting, rash, photosensitivity

Drug	Trade name	Preparation	Strength	Conditions and doses	Comments	Side-effects
Itraconazole	Sporanox	Capsule Oral liquid	100mg 10mg/ml	Pityriasis versicolor: 200mg/d for 7 days; tinea corporis and cruris: 100mg/d for 15 days or 200mg/d for 7 days; tinea pedis and manuum: 100mg/d for 30 days or 200mg 2 times/d for 7 days; onychomycosis: 200mg/d for 3 months or pulses of 200mg 2 times/d for 7 days repeated after 21 day interval	Caution in hepatic disease, renal impairment, congestive heart failure, pregnancy, breast feeding	Nausea, abdominal pain, dyspepsia, constipation, headache, dizziness, raised liver enzymes, menstrual disorders
Ketoconazole	Nizoral	Tablet	200mg	Resistant dermatophyte infections of skin and finger nails: 200mg/d for 14 days (max 400mg/d)	Contraindicated in hepatic impairment (monitor liver function), porphyria, pregnancy, breast feeding	Nausea, vomiting, abdominal pain, headache, rash, urticaria, pruritus
Terbinafine	Lamisil	Tablet	250mg	Tinea pedis, cruris and corporis, onychomycosis: 250mg/d for 2 weeks to 3 months	Caution in hepatic and renal impairment, pregnancy, breast feeding, psoriasis	Abdominal discomfort, anorexia, nausea, diarrhoea, headache, rash, urticaria

Topical antiviral preparations

Drug	Trade name	Preparation	Strength	Conditions and doses	Comments	Side-effects
Aciclovir	Zovirax	Cream	5%	Herpes simplex infection: apply 5 times/d for 5–10 days starting at first signs of attack	Caution to avoid contact with eyes and mucous membranes; may be used with systemic antivirals for deeper infections	Transient stinging or burning, occasionally erythema, itching or drying of skin
Penciclovir	Vectavir	Cream	1%	Herpes simplex infection: apply every 2h during waking hours for 4 days starting at first signs of attack	Caution to avoid contact with eyes and mucous membranes; may be used with systemic antivirals for deeper infections	Transient stinging, burning and numbness

Oral antifungal preparations

Drug	Trade name	Preparation	Strength	Conditions and doses	Comments	Side-effects
Aciclovir	Generic	Tablet	200mg, 400mg, 800mg	Herpes simplex infection, treatment: 200mg 5 times/d for 5 days; prevention of recurrence: 200mg 4 times/d or 400mg 2 times/d interrupted every 6–12 months; herpes zoster: 800mg 5 times/d for 7 days	Caution in renal impairment (maintain adequate hydration), pregnancy, breast feeding	Nausea, vomiting, abdominal pain, diarrhoea, headache, fatigue, rash, urticaria, pruritus, photosensitivity
	Zovirax	Tablet	200mg, 400mg, 800mg			
		Suspension	200mg/5ml, 400mg/5ml			
Famciclovir	Famvir	Tablet	125mg, 250mg, 500mg, 750mg	Herpes zoster: 250mg 3 times/d for 7 days or 750mg/d for 7 days	Caution in renal impairment, pregnancy, breast feeding	Nausea, vomiting, headache, dizziness, confusion, hallucinations, rash
Valaciclovir	Valtrex	Tablet	500mg	Herpes simplex, first and recurrent infections: 500mg 2 times/d for 5 days; herpes zoster: 1g 3 times/d for 7 days	Caution in renal impairment (maintain adequate hydration), pregnancy, breast feeding	Nausea, vomiting, abdominal pain, diarrhoea, headache, fatigue, rash, urticaria, pruritus, photosensitivity

Parasiticidal preparations

Drug	Trade name	Preparation	Strength	Conditions and doses	Comments	Side-effects
Carbaryl	Carylderm	Liquid	1% (aqueous)	*Head lice:* rub into dry hair and scalp allow to dry naturally shampoo after 12h and comb wet hair; do not use more than once weekly for 3 consecutive weeks	Caution to avoid contact with eyes and broken skin; use aqueous solutions in people with asthma and eczema	Skin irritation
		Lotion	0.5% (alcoholic)			
Malathion	Derbac M	Liquid	0.5% (aqueous)	*Head lice:* rub 0.5% preparation into dry hair and scalp allow to dry naturally and shampoo after 12h or apply 1% shampoo to wet hair and rinse after 5min and repeat twice at intervals of 3 days; *Crab lice:* apply 0.5% aqueous preparation over whole body allow to dry naturally and wash off after 12h; *Scabies:* apply 0.5% preparation over whole body and wash off after 24h	Caution to avoid contact with eyes and broken skin; use aqueous solutions for head lice and scabies in people with asthma and eczema	Skin irritation
	Prioderm	Lotion	0.5% (alcoholic)			
	Quellada M	Liquid	0.5% (aqueous)			
		Cream shampoo	1%			
Permethrin	Lyclear Creme Rinse	Cream rinse	1%	*Head lice:* apply to clean damp hair and rinse after 10min *Scabies:* apply over whole body and wash off after 8–12h; *Crab lice:* apply to whole body and wash off after 12h	Caution to avoid contact with eyes and broken skin	Pruritus, erythema, stinging, rashes, oedema (rare)
	Lyclear Dermal Cream	Cream	5%			
Phenothrin	Full Marks	Liquid	0.5% (aqueous)	*Head lice:* apply 0.5% aqueous preparation to dry hair allow to dry naturally and shampoo after 12h or apply 0.2% alcoholic preparation to dry hair allow to dry naturally and shampoo after 2h or apply mousse to dry hair and shampoo after 30min; *Crab lice:* apply 0.2% alcoholic preparation to whole body and wash off after 12h; do not use more than once weekly for 3 consecutive weeks	Caution to avoid contact with eyes and broken skin; use aqueous solutions for head lice and scabies in people with asthma and eczema	Skin irritation
		Lotion	0.2% (alcoholic)			
		Mousse	0.5% (alcoholic)			

Abbreviations

ACE	Angiotensin converting enzyme
AIDS	Acquired immune deficiency syndrome
ECG	Electrocardiogram
ESR	Erythrocyte sedimentation rate
GP	General practitioner
H1-receptor	Histamine type 1 receptor
H2-receptor	Histamine type 2 receptor
HAART	Highly active antiretroviral therapy
HIV	Human immunodeficiency virus
HLA	Human leukocyte antigen
HPV	Human papilloma virus
HSV-1	Herpes simplex virus type 1
HSV-2	Herpes simplex virus type 2
Ig	Immunoglobulin
MCV1	Molluscum contagiosum virus type 1
MCV2	Molluscum contagiosum virus type 2
NSAID	Non-steroidal anti-inflammatory drug
PUVA	Psoralens ultraviolet A
RAST	Radioallergosorbent
spp	Species
UV	Ultraviolet
UVA	Ultraviolet type A
UVB	Ultraviolet type B

USEFUL ADDRESSES AND WEBSITES

For health professionals

Action on Dermatology

Web: www.modern.nhs.uk/scripts/default.asp?site_id=30&id=2712

Part of the National Patients Access Team. Action on Dermatology aims to improve access to services for patients by identifying areas of best practice. There are currently 16 pilot sites looking at the delivery of dermatology services.

American Academy of Dermatology

PO Box 4014, Schaumburg, IL 60168-4014, USA

Tel: (+1) 847 330 0230
Fax: (+1) 847 330 0050
Web: www.aad.org/

Represents practising dermatologists in the United States. Website contains resources for continuing medical education.

British Association of Dermatologists

19 Fitzroy Square, London, W1T 6EH, UK

Tel: +44 (0) 207 383 0266
Fax: +44 (0) 207 388 5263
Email: admin@bad.org.uk
Web: www.bad.org.uk

Information for health professionals who want to know more about dermatology and its practice, including information on training and careers, and guidelines prepared by the British Association of Dermatologists and the Royal College of General Practitioners.

Cochrane Skin Group

Web: www.nottingham.ac.uk/%7Emuzd/index.htm

An international network of people committed to producing and updating reviews of trials relating to skin conditions. Part of the Cochrane Collaboration.

DermIS

Web: dermis.multimedica.de/index_e.htm

International portal for dermatology, including an online image atlas and information system. Produced by the Department of Clinical Social Medicine (University of Heidelberg) and the Department of Dermatology (University of Erlangen).

Evidence-Based Dermatology
David A. Barzilai, Founder and Co-Chief Editor, Case Western, Reserve University, Cleveland, Ohio, USA

Email: dxb69@po.cwru.edu
Web: www.ebderm.org

Web resources in evidence-based medicine, epidemiology, and health services research for dermatologists and skin researchers.

History of Dermatology Society
President: Lawrence Charles Parish, MD
1819 J. F. Kennedy Boulevard, Philadelphia, PA 19103, USA

Tel: (+1) 215 563 8333
Fax: (+1) 215 563 3044
E-mail: Lawrence.Parish@mail.tju.edu
Web: www.dermato.med.br/hds/

Founded to promote an understanding of the development of the specialty of dermatology. The Society holds annual meetings at the time of the American Academy of Dermatology and an extraordinary session during the International Congress of Dermatology.

International Skin Care Nursing Group
School of Nursing and Midwifery, Nightingale Building, Highfield, Southampton, SO17 1BJ, UK

Tel: +44 (0) 238 059 8236
Fax: +44 (0) 238 059 7900
Web: www.soton.ac.uk/~isng/

Aims to raise the profile of skin health and the contribution that nurses can make in this area of health care.

Primary Care Dermatology Society

Gable House, 40 High Street, Rickmansworth, Hertfordshire, WD3 1ER, UK

Tel: +44 (0) 1923 711 678
Email: pcds@pcds.org.uk
Web: www.pcds.org.uk

Forum for GPs to exchange views on primary care dermatology, develop skills and progress clinical research.

Referral advice: a guide to appropriate referral from general to specialist services. 2001.

National Institute for Clinical Excellence,
MidCity Place, 71 High Holborn, London, WC1V 6NA, UK

Tel: +44 (0) 207 067 5800
Fax: +44 (0) 207 067 5801
Web: www.nice.org.uk/cat.asp?c=1042

Provides advice on prioritizing the referral of patients from primary care to specialist services. It also gives specific recommendations on how soon the patient should be seen by specialist services.

Skin Therapy Letter

Web: stl.skincareguide.com/tf/content.asp?z=400

International publication for dermatologists. It is evidence based, and written by world-renowned dermatology opinion leaders.

For patients
Acne Support Group

PO Box 9, Newquay, Cornwall, TR9 6WG, UK

Tel: +44 (0) 870 870 2263
Web: www.m2w3.com/acne/

Advice and information for people with acne.

British Association of Dermatologists

19 Fitzroy Square, London, W1T 6EH, UK

Tel: +44 (0) 207 383 0266

Fax: +44 (0) 207 388 5263
Email: admin@bad.org.uk
Web: www.bad.org.uk

Information on skin and skin diseases, prepared by UK dermatologists.
Patients can find out what a dermatologist does and how to find the
help they need. Lists support groups for people with skin disorders.

Bullous Pemphigoid Support Group
17 Barley Mount, Redhills, Exeter, EX4 1RP, UK

CancerBACUP
3 Bath Place, Rivington Street, London, EC2A 3DR, UK

Tel: Freephone 0808 800 1234
Fax: +44 (0) 207 696 9002
Web: www.cancerbacup.org.uk

Provides high-quality and up-to-date information, practical advice and
support for cancer patients and their families.

Cancer Research UK
PO Box 123, Lincoln's Inn Fields, London, WC2A 3PX, UK

Tel: +44 (0) 207 242 0200
Specialist information nurses: +44 (0) 207 269 3142
Fax: +44 (0) 207 269 3100
Web: www.cancerresearchuk.org

Dedicated to research on the causes, treatment and prevention of cancer.

Congenital Melanocytic Naevus Support Group
Bridge Chapel Centre, Heath Road, Garston, Liverpool, L19 4XR, UK

Tel: +44 (0) 151 281 9716
Fax: +44 (0) 151 281 9717

Hairline International, The Alopecia Patients' Society
Lyons Court, 1668 High Street, Knowle, West Midlands, B93 0LY, UK
(Enclose an A4 SAE)

Tel: +44 (0) 1564 775 281
Fax: +44 (0) 1564 782 270

Herpes Viruses Association

41 North Road, London, N7 9DP, UK

Tel: +44 (0) 207 607 9661 (office and Minicom V)
Tel: +44 (0) 207 609 9061 (helpline - 24 hours access).
Web: www.herpes.org.uk

Advice and information for people with genital herpes simplex and shingles.

Ichthyosis Support Group

PO Box 7913, Reading, RG6 4ZQ, UK

Tel/fax: +44 (0) 207 461 9034
Email: isg@ichthyosis.org.uk
Web: www.ichthyosis.co.uk

National contact for people with ichthyosis and their carers.

LUPUS UK

St James House, Eastern Road, Romford, Essex, RMI 3NH, UK

Tel: +44 (0) 1708 731 251 (5 lines) and 24 hour answerphone
Fax: +44 (0) 1708 731 252
Email: headoffice@lupus-uk.freeserve.co.uk
Web: www.lupusuk.com

For people with systemic lupus erythematosus.

National Eczema Society

Hill House, Highgate Hill, London, N19 5NA, UK

Tel: +44 (0) 207 281 3553
Eczema Help Line: +44 (0) 870 241 3604
Fax: +44 (0) 207 281 6395
Web: www.eczema.org/

Information and advice service for people with eczema and their carers.

National Lichen Sclerosus Support Group

PO Box 7600, Hungerford, Berkshire, RG17 7XD, UK
(Enclose SAE for reply).

Web: www.lichensclerosus.org

Support and self-help information for people with lichen sclerosus.

Psoriasis Association

Milton House, 7 Milton Street, Northampton, NN2 7JG, UK

Tel: +44 (0) 1604 711 129
Fax: +44 (0) 1604 792 894
Email: mail@psoriasis.demon.co.uk
Web: www.psoriasis-association.org.uk

Support and information for people with psoriasis.

Skin Care Campaign

Web: www.skincarecampaign.org/

Umbrella organization representing the interests of people with skin diseases in the UK.

The Vitiligo Society

125 Kennington Road, London, SE11 6SF

Tel: +44 (0) 207 840 0855
Email: all@vitiligosociety.org.uk
Web: www.vitiligosociety.org.uk/

Offers support and understanding to people with vitiligo and campaigns for a better understanding among the medical profession and the general public of how it feels to live with vitiligo.

References

Acne

1. Layton AM. Optimal management of acne to prevent scarring and psychological sequelae. *Am J Clin Dermatol* 2001;2:135–41.
2. Garner SE, Eady EA, Popesccu C, et al. Minocycline for acne vulgaris: efficacy and safety (Cochrane Review). Cochrane Database Syst Rev 2003;(1):CD002086.
3. Jacobs DG, Deutsch NL, Brewer M. Suicide, depression, and isotretinoin: is there a causal link? *J Am Acad Dermatol* 2001;45:S168–75.
4. Altman RS, Altman LJ, Altman JS. A proposed set of guidelines for routine blood tests during isotretinoin therapy for acne vulgaris. *Dermatology* 2002;204:232–5.

Actinic keratosis

1. Frost C, Green A. Epidemiology of solar keratoses. *Br J Dermatol* 1994;131:455–64.
2. Epstein E. Does intermittent "pulse" topical 5-fluorouracil therapy allow destruction of actinic keratoses without significant inflammation? *J Amer Acad Dermatol* 1998;38:77–80.

Alopecia areata

1. Sinclair RD, Banfield CC, Dawber RPR. Handbook of Diseases of the Hair and Scalp. Oxford: Blackwell Science, 1999:75–84.
2. MacDonald Hull SP, Wood ML, Hutchinson PE, et al. Guidelines for the management of alopecia areata. *Br J Dermatol* 2003;149:692–9.

Basal cell carcinoma

1. Telfer NR, Colver GB, Bowers PW. Guidelines for the management of basal cell carcinoma. *Br J Dermatol* 1999;141:415–23.
2. Bath FJ, Bong J, Perkins W, Williams HC. Interventions for basal cell carcinoma of the skin (Cochrane Review). In: The Cochrane Library, Issue 2, 2003. Oxford: Update Software.

Bowen's disease

1. Eedy D, Gavin G. Thirteen year retrospective study of Bowen's disease in Northern Ireland. *Br J Dermatol* 1987;117:715–20.
2. Cox N, Eedy D, Morton C. Guidelines for management of Bowen's disease. *Br J Dermatol* 1999;141:633–41.

Candidiasis

1. Rex JH, Walsh TJ, Sobel JD, et al. Practice guidelines for the treatment of candidiasis. *Clin Infect Dis* 2000;30:662–78.

Dermatophyte infections

1. Fuller LC, Child FJ, Midgley G, et al. Diagnosis and management of scalp ringworm. *BMJ* 2003;326:539–41.
2. Higgins EM, Fuller LC, Smith CH. Guidelines for the management of tinea capitis. British Association of Dermatologists. *Br J Dermatol* 2000;143:53–8.
3. Bell-Syer SEM, Hart R, Crawford F, Togerson DJ, Tyrrell W, Russell I. Oral treatments for fungal infections of the skin of the foot (Cochrane Review).In: The Cochrane library, Issue 1, 2003. Oxford: Update Software.
4. Roberts DT, Taylor WD, Boyle J. Guidelines for treatment of onychomycosis. *Br J Dermatol* 2003;148:402–10.

Discoid lupus erythematosus

1. Jessop S, Whitelaw D, Jordaan F. Drugs for discoid lupus erythematosus (Cochrane Review). In: The Cochrane Library, Issue 1, 2003. Oxford: Update Software.

Eczema/dermatitis

Atopic eczema

1. Bleiker TO, Shahidullah H, Dutton E, et al. The prevalence and incidence of atopic dermatitis in a birth cohort: The importance of a family history of atopy. *Arch Dermatol* 2000;136:274.
2. McHenry PM, Williams HC, Bingham EA. Management of atopic eczema. Joint Workshop of the British Association of Dermatologists and the Research Unit of the Royal College of Physicians of London. *BMJ* 1995;310:843–7.

Contact dermatitis

1. Rietschel RL, Fowler JF, Jr. Fisher's contact dermatitis. Fifth edition. Philadelphia: Lippincott, Williams and Wilkins, 2001.
2. Bourke J, Coulson I, English J. Guidelines for care of contact dermatitis. *Br J Dermatol* 2001;145:877–85.

Seborrhoeic eczema

1. Carr MM, Pryce DM, Ive FA. Treatment of seborrhoeic dermatitis with ketoconazole: I Response of the scalp to topical ketoconazole. *Br J Dermatol* 1987;116:213–6.
2. Green CA, Farr PM, Shuster S. Treatment of seborrhoeic dermatitis with ketoconazole: II Response of the seborrhoeic dermatitis of the face, scalp and trunk to topical ketoconazole. *Br J Dermatol* 1987;116:217–221.

Erysipelas

1. Bonnetblanc JM, Bedane C. Erysipelas: recognition and management. *Am J Clin Dermatol* 2003;4:157–63.
2. Badger C, Seers K, Preston N, et al. Antibiotics/anti-inflammatories for reducing acute inflammatory episodes in lymphoedema of the limbs (Protocol for a Cochrane review). In: The Cochrane Library, Issue 1, 2003. Oxford: Update Software.

Head lice

1. Dodd CS. Interventions for treating headlice (Cochrane Review). In: The Cochrane library, Issue 1, 2003. Oxford: Update Software.

Herpes simplex

1. Bacon TH, Levin MJ, Leary JJ, et al. Herpes simplex virus resistant to acyclovir and penciclovir after two decades of antiviral therapy. *Clin Microbiol Rev* 2003;16:114–28.

Ichthyosis

1. DiGiovanna JJ, Robinson-Bostom L. Ichthyosis: etiology, diagnosis and management. *Am J Clin Dermatol* 2003;4:81–95.
2. Compton JG, DiGiovanna JJ, Johnston KA, et al. Mapping of the associated phenotype of an absent granular layer in ichthyosis vulgaris to the epidermal differentiation complex on chromosome 1. *Exp Dermatol* 2002;11:518–26.
3. Holden C, English J, Jordan A, et al. Advised best practice for the use of emollients in eczema and other dry skin conditions. *J Dermatolog Treat* 2002;13:103–6.

Impetigo

1. McCormick A, Fleming D, Charlton J. Morbidity Studies from General Practice. Fourth National Study, 1991–2. London: HMSO, 1995.
2. Luby S, Agboatwalla M, Schnell BM, et al. The effect of an antibacterial soap on impetigo incidence, Karachi, Pakistan. *Am J Trop Med Hyg* 2002:67:430–5.
3. Koning S, Verhagen AP, van Suijlekom-Smit LWA, et al. Interventions for impetigo (Protocol for a Cochrane Review). In: The Cochrane Library, Issue 1, 2003. Oxford: Update Software.

Lichen planus

1. Graham-Brown RAC. Lichen planus. In: New Clinical Applications in Dermatology III. (Verbov J, ed). London: Kluwer Academic Publications, 1988:53–77.

2. Chan ES-Y, Thornhill M, Zakrzewska J. Interventions for treating oral lichen planus (Cochrane Review). In: The Cochrane Library, Issue 2, 2003. Oxford: Update Software.

Melanoma (malignant)

1. Melia J, Moss C, Graham-Brown R, et al. The relation between mortality from malignant melanoma and early detection in the Cancer Research Campaign Mole watcher Study. *Br J Cancer* 2001;85:803–7.
2. Roberts DLL, Anstey AV, Barlow RJ, Cox NH on behalf of the British Association of Dermatologists, and Newton Bishop JA, Corrie PG, Evans J, et al on behalf of the Melanoma Study Group. UK guidelines for the management of cutaneous melanoma. *Br J Dermatol* 2002;146:7–17.

Pemphigoid

1. Cooper SM, Wojnarowska F. Treatments of choice for bullous pemphigoid. *Skin Therapy Lett* 2002;7:4–6.
2. Wojnarowska F, Kirtschig G, Highet A, et al. Guidelines for the management of bullous pemphigoid. *Br J Dermatol* 2002; 147:214–21.
3. Joly P, Roujeau JC, Benichou J, et al. A comparison of oral and topical corticosteroids in patients with bullous pemphigoid. *N Engl J Med* 2002;346:321–7.

Photosensitivity

1. Roelandts R. The diagnosis of photosensitivity. *Arch Dermatol* 2000;136:1152–7.

Pityriasis versicolor

1. Kose O, Bulent Tastan H, et al. Comparison of a single 400mg dose versus a 7-day 200mg daily dose of itraconazole in the treatment of tinea versicolor. *J Dermatolog Treat* 2002;13:77–9.

Pruritus (generalized)

1. Savin JA. How should we define itching? *J Am Acad Dermatol* 1998;38:268–9.
2. Twycross R, Greaves MW, Handwerker H, et al. Itch: scratching more than the surface. *Q J Med* 2003;96:7–26.

Psoriasis

1. Camp RDR. Psoriasis. In: Textbook of Dermatology (6th edition). (Champion RH, Burton JL, Burns DA, Breathnach SM, eds). Oxford: Blackwell Science, 1998:1589–649.

Rosacea

1. Wilkin J, Dahl M, Detmar M, et al. Standard classification of rosacea. *J Am Acad Dermatol* 2002;46:584–7.
2. Szlachcic A. The link between Helicobacter pylori infection and rosacea. *J Eur Acad Dermatol Venereol* 2002;16:228–333.
3. Bogetti P, Boltri M, Spagnoli G, et al. Surgical treatment of rhinophyma: a comparison of techniques. *Aesthetic Plast Surg* 2002;26:57–60.

Scabies

1. Lacarrubba F, Musumeci ML, Caltabiano R, et al. High-magnification videodermatoscopy: a new non-invasive diagnostic tool for scabies in children. *Paediatr Dermatol* 2001;18:439–41.
2. Obasanjo OO, Wu P, Conlon M, et al. An outbreak of scabies in a teaching hospital: lessons learned. *Infect Control Hosp Epidemiol* 2001;22:13–18.
3. The management of scabies. *Drug Ther Bull* 2002;40:43–6.
4. Wendel K, Rompalo A. Scabies and pediculosis pubis: an update of treatment regimens and general review. *Clin Infect Dis* 2002;35(Suppl 2):S146–51.
5. Scott GR. European guideline for the management of scabies. *Int J STD AIDS* 2001;12(Suppl 3):58–61.
6. Vaidhyanathan U. Review of ivermectin in scabies. *J Cutan Med Surg* 2001;5:496–504.
7. Chouela E, Abeldano A, Pellerano G, et al. Diagnosis and treatment of scabies: a practical guide. *Am J Clin Dermatol* 2002;3:9–18.

Squamous cell carcinoma

1. Preston DS, Stern RS. Nonmelanoma cancers of the skin. *N Engl J Med* 1992;327:1649–62.
2. Boyle J, Mackie RM, Briggs JD, et al. Cancer, warts and sunshine in renal transplant patients. *Lancet* 1984;i:702–5.
3. Liddingtin M, Richardson AJ, Higgins RM, et al. Skin cancer in renal transplant recipients. *Br J Surg* 1989;76:1002–5.
4. Motley R, Kersey P, Lawrence C, on behalf of the British Association of Dermatologists, the British Association of Plastic Surgeons and the Faculty of Clinical Oncology of the Royal

College of Radiologists. Multiprofessional guidelines for the management of the patient with primary cutaneous squamous cell carcinoma. *Br J Dermatol* 2002;146:18–25.

Urticaria and angio-oedema

1. Kozel MM, Mekkes JR, Bossuyt PMM, et al. The effectiveness of a history-based diagnostic approach in chronic urticaria and angio-oedema. *Arch Dermatology* 1998;134:1575–80.
2. Grattan C, Powell S, Humphreys F. Management and diagnostic guidelines for urticaria and angio-oedema. *Br J Dermatol* 2001;144:708–14.
3. Humphreys F, Hunter JAA. The characteristics of urticaria in 390 patients. *Br J Dermatol* 1998;138:635–8.

Vasculitis

1. Stadler R, Ruszczak Z. Therapeutic guidelines in vasculitis. *Int Angiol* 1995;14:188–96.
2. Lotti T, Ghersetich I, Comacchi C, et al. Cutaneous small vessel vasculitis. *J Am Acad Dermatol* 2003;39:667–87

Venous ulcers

1. Mekkes JR, Loots MAM, Van Der Wal AC, et al. Causes, investigation and treatment of leg ulceration. *Br J Dermatol* 2003;148:388–401.
2. Cullum N, Nelson EA, Fletcher AW, et al. Compression for venous leg ulcers (Cochrane Review). In: The Cochrane Library, Issue 1, 2003. Oxford: Update Software.
3. Bradley M, Cullum N, Nelson EA, et al. Systematic reviews of wound care management: (2) dressings and topical agents used in the healing of chronic wounds. *Health Techn Assess* 1999;3:1–135.
4. Palfreyman SJ, Michaels JA, Lochiel R, et al. Dressings for venous leg ulcers (Protocol for a Cochrane Review). In: The Cochrane library, Issue 1, 2003. Oxford: Update Software.

Vitiligo

1. Njoo MD, Spuls PI, Bos JD, et al. Nonsurgical repigmentation therapies in vitiligo. Meta-analysis of the literature. *Arch Dermatol* 1998;134:1532–40.
2. Barrett C, Whitton M. Interventions for vitiligo (Protocol for a Cochrane Review). In: The Cochrane Library, Issue 2, 2003. Oxford: Update Software.

Warts (viral)

1. Gibbs S, Harvey I, Sterling J, et al. Local treatments for cutaneous warts. *BMJ* 2002;325:461.
2. Sterling JC, Handfield-Jones S, Hudson P. Guidelines for the treatment of cutaneous warts. *Br J Dermatol* 2001;144:4–11.
3. Maw R, von Krogh G. The management of anal warts. *BMJ* 2000;321:910–1.
4. Leman JA, Benton EC. Verrucas. Guidelines for management. *Am J Clin Dermatol* 2000;1:143–9.

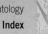

Index

Note: Please note that page numbers followed by "f" or "t" denote figures and tables respectively, those followed by "cs" represent case studies.

A

aciclovir, 148t, 149t
  herpes simplex, 54
acitretin, 138t
  discoid lupus erythematosus, 32
acne, 8–15
  aetiology, 8–9
  diagnosis, 9–10
  differential diagnosis, 10f
  epidemiology, 8
  excoriated, 20f
  prevention, 11
  subtypes, 10t
  treatment, 11–15, 11f, 12f, 13f
  typical lesions, 8f, 9f
acne rosacea *see* rosacea
acral melanoma, 67
actinic dermatitis, 78
actinic keratosis, 15–16
  aetiology, 15
  diagnosis, 15–16
  epidemiology, 15
  prevention, 16
  squamous cell carcinoma *vs.*, 16
  treatment, 16, 16f, 17f
adapalene, 12f, 139t
Addison's disease, 25
addresses, 152–157
adrenaline, 104–105
Aknemin, 142t
Aknemycin Plus, 140t
alclometasone diproprionate, 128t
alcohol-based lotions, head lice, 51
alcohol intake, discoid eczema, 42
allergy/allergens
  atopic eczema, 33–34
  contact dermatitis, 38f, 39, 41
  testing, 41, 102, 103
  urticaria, 102, 103
alopecia areata, 17–19, 19f
  aetiology, 18
  diagnosis, 18
  treatment, 18–19
alopecia totalis, 18
alopecia universalis, 18

Alphaderm, 133t
Alphosyl, 136t
aminoglycosides, 40f
Anabact, 145t
androgens, acne, 9
angio-oedema, 99–105
  causes, 102f
  classifications, 100f
  diagnosis, 100–103
  epidemiology, 100
anogenital warts, 114
  treatment, 118
antibiotics
  acne, 12–13
  eczema/dermatitis, 37
  rosacea, 92
anticoagulants, erysipelas, 48
antihistamines
  eczema, 37f
  urticaria, 104
antipruritic agents, 84
antiseptics, impetigo treatment, 58
antiviral drugs, 148t, 149t
  herpes simplex infection, 54
  see also specific drugs
artefactual skin disease, 19, 20f, 21f
arthropathic psoriasis, 87, 88f
atopic eczema, 33–35, 33f
  aetiology, 34
  definition, 33f
  diagnosis, 35
  epidemiology, 33–34, 33f
  lichen simplex, 62
  prevention, 35
  treatment, 35–38
atypical mole syndrome, 121–122cs,
  121f, 122f
autoimmune disease
  alopecia areata, 18
  discoid lupus erythematosus, 32
  lichen planus and, 59
  pemphigoid, 73–75
  vitiligo, 111
  see also specific disorders
AVOCA, 143t

azaleic acid, 12f, 139t
azathioprine, pemphigoid, 75
azoles, seborrhoeic eczema, 44

B

bacterial infections, 56
  acne, 9
  erysipelas, 46
  folliculitis, acne *vs.*, 10
  impetigo, 56–57, 57f
  see also antibiotics; *specific infections*
Bactroban, 145t
basal cell carcinoma, 21–23, 21f
  clinical variants, 22f
  diagnosis, 22
  epidemiology, 21
  treatment, 22–23
Behçet's disease, 106f
benzoyl peroxide, 12f, 139t
Betacap, 129t
betamethasone, 129t, 136t
Betta-mousse, 129t
Betnovate, 129t
biopsy/excision
  actinic keratosis, 16f, 17f
  malignant melanoma, 69
  melanocytic naevi, 65
  pemphigoid blister, 74
blistering, pemphigoid, 73–75
blue naevus, 64f
Bowen's disease, 23–24, 24f
  prevention, 23
  treatment, 24
Brevoxyl, 139t

C

calcineurin antagonists, eczema, 37f
calcipotriol, 136t
  vitiligo, 112
Calmurid, 133t
Candida albicans infection, 24–25
candidal intertrigo, 25f
candidiasis, 24–25
  aetiology, 24–25
  mucocutaneous, 25, 25f
  treatment, 26f
Canesten, 133t, 146t
carbaryl, 50, 150t
Carbo-Dome, 136t
carcinomas *see* basal cell carcinoma;
  squamous cell carcinoma

Carylderm, 150t
case studies
  atypical mole syndrome and
    melanoma, 121–122, 121f, 122f
  contact dermatitis and secondary
    tinea pedis, 125–126, 125f, 126f
  lichen planus and NSAID use,
    123–124, 123f, 124f
  psoriasis, 119–120, 120f
cellulitis, 48
chemical burns, artefactual, 21f
children
  atopic eczema, 34
  head lice, 48
  impetigo, 56
  molluscum contagiosum, 70, 71
chlorpheniramine, 104
chromates, 40f
ciclosporin, 138t
  psoriasis, 89f
cimetidine, urticaria, 104
clindamycin, 12f, 139t
Clinitar, 136t
clioquinol, 129t, 132t, 134t
clobetasol butyrate, 130t
clobetasol propionate, 130t
clotrimazole, 128t, 133t, 146t
coal tar, 136t
cobalt, contact dermatitis, 40f
cockarde naevus, 64f
Cocois, 136t
co-cyprindiol, 13, 141t
coldsores *see* herpes simplex infection
colophony, 40f
combs, head lice, 51
condoms, 54
contact dermatitis, 38–42
  aetiology, 39, 40f
  allergic, 38f, 39
  diagnosis, 41
  epidemiology, 38
  irritant, 38f, 39
  prevention, 41
  secondary tinea pedis, 125–126cs,
    125f, 126f
  treatment, 42
corticosteroids, 128–135t
  alopecia areata, 18–19
  atopic eczema, 37f
  contact dermatitis induction, 40f
  discoid eczema, 42

discoid lupus erythematosus, 32
  eczema/dermatitis, 36, 37f, 40f,
    42, 44, 45
  lichen planus, 62
  pemphigoid, 75
  psoriasis, 89f
  seborrhoeic eczema, 44
  urticaria, 104
  varicose (stasis) eczema, 45
  vitiligo, 112
crotamiton, 133t
crusted (Norwegian) scabies, 95
cryotherapy
  basal cell carcinoma, 23
  molluscum contagiosum, 70
  warts (viral), 115, 117f, 118
Cuplex, 143t
Curatoderm, 137t
curettage
  actinic keratosis, 16f, 17f
  basal cell carcinoma, 23
  warts, 117f
cutaneous lupus erythematosus *see*
  discoid lupus erythematosus
cutaneous vasculitis *see* vasculitis
Cutivate, 132t
cyproterone, 141t

D

Daktacort, 133t
Daktarin, 146t
Dalacin T, 139t
delusions of parasitosis, 20f
Dennie–Morgan infraorbital fold, 35
depression, isotretinoin, 14
Derbac M, 150t
dermatitis *see* eczema/dermatitis
dermatitis artefacta, 20f
dermatofibroma (histiocytoma),
  25–27
  diagnosis, 26–27
  epidemiology, 26
dermatological pathomimicry, 20f
dermatophyte infections, 27–29, 27f
  aetiology, 28–29
  diagnosis and management, 28f, 29
  epidemiology, 27–28
  nails, 30f
  scalp, 28f
  see also specific infections

dermatoscopy
  malignant melanoma, 68
  scabies, 95
Dermovate, 130t
desoximetasone, 130t
Dianette, 141t
diclofenac, 143t
  actinic keratosis, 16f, 17f
diet, manipulation, 11, 38
Differin, 139t
Diflucan, 147t
diflucortolone valerate, 131t
Dioderm, 133t
diphencyprone, alopecia areata, 19
Diprosalic, 128t
Diprosone, 128t
discoid eczema, 42–43, 42f
discoid lupus erythematosus, 31–32,
  31f
  aetiology, 31
  diagnosis, 32
  epidemiology, 31
  photosensitivity, 78
  treatment, 32
dithranol, 137t
  psoriasis, 89f
Dithro-cream, 137t
Doppler ankle brachial pressure
  index, 109
Dovobet, 136t
Dovonex, 136t
doxepin cream, 134t
  pruritus, 82
doxepine, pruritus, 84
doxycycline, 141t
dressings, habituations, 20f
drug-induced conditions
  acne, 10f
  contact dermatitis, 40f
  lichen planus, 60, 123–124cs,
    123f, 124f
  pruritus, 83f
  urticaria, 103f
drugs
  acne treatment, 12–14, 13f
  photosensitivity, 78
  topical *see* topical treatments
  see also individual drugs/drug types
dry skin, 35
Duofilm, 143t

E

ear, painful nodules, 72, 73f
Econacort, 133t
econazole, 133t, 146t
Ecostatin, 146t
eczema/dermatitis, 33–47
    actinic dermatitis, 78
    antibiotics, 37
    antihistamines, 37f
    artefactual, 20f
    atopic *see* atopic eczema
    contact *see* contact dermatitis
    discoid eczema, 42–43, 42f
    eczema herpeticum, 35, 38
    infections, 36–37
    photocontact dermatitis, 78
    seborrhoeic eczema, 34f, 43–44,
        43f, 79
    varicose (stasis) eczema, 44–46
    see also individual types
eczema herpeticum, 35, 36f, 38
Efcortelan, 133t
Efudix, 143t
elderly, pemphigoid, 73
Elidel, 135t
Elocon, 134t
emollients, 127f
    bath additives, 127f
    eczema, 36, 37f
    ichthyosis, 55
    pruritus, 82
    psoriasis, 89f
endocrine disorders
    Addison's disease, 25
    pruritus induction, 83f
environmental factors
    atopic eczema, 34
    manipulation, 37f, 38
Erymax, 141t
erysipelas, 46–48, 46f
    aetiology, 47
    diagnosis, 47–48
    differential diagnosis, 48
    epidemiology, 46–47
    predisposing factors, 47f
    treatment, 48
erythema nodosum, 105
erythematous papules, acne, 9f
erythrodermic psoriasis, 87
erythromycin, 12f, 13, 139t, 141t
    erysipelas, 48
erythroplasia of Queyrat, 23

erythropoietic protoporphyria, 77
ethinylestradiol (co-cyprindiol), 141t
Eumovate, 130t
Eurax, 133t
'exclamation mark hairs,' 18, 19f
Exelderm, 147t
Exorex, 136t
eye involvement, rosacea, 92

F

facial milia, acne *vs.,* 10
famciclovir, 149t
Famvir, 149t
fever, erysipelas, 46f
finasteride, 144t
flexural psoriasis, 86
fluconazole, 147t
fludroxycortide (flurandrenolone),
    131t
fluocinolone acetonide, 132t
fluocinolone propionate, 132t
5-fluorouracil, 143t
    actinic keratosis, 16f, 17f
    basal cell carcinoma, 23
follicular lichen planus, 61
formaldehyde, 40f, 142t
Forte, 131t
Fucibet, 129t
Fucidin, 133t, 145t
Full Marks, 150t
fungal infections, 79–80
    Candida albicans, 24–25
    seborrhoeic eczema, 43
fusidic acid, 129t, 133t, 145t
    impetigo treatment, 58

G

genetic factors
    acne, 8
    alopecia areata, 18
    atopic eczema, 34
    ichthyosis, 55
    psoriasis, 85
genital candidiasis, 25f
genital herpes, 53–54
gingivitis, 60
glutaraldehyde, 142t
Glutarol, 142t
granuloma, pyogenic, 90–91, 90f
griseofulvin, 27, 147t
Grisovin, 147t
guttate psoriasis, 85–86

H

H1-receptor antagonists, 84
Haelan, 131t
hair
   lichen planus, 60–61
   loss, 17–19
      see also alopecia areata
   pulling habit, 20f
halo naevus, 64f
head lice, 48–51
   aetiology, 49
   characteristics, 49f
   diagnosis, 50
   differential diagnosis, 50f
   epidemiology, 48–49
   life cycle, 49f
   prevention, 50
   treatment, 50–51
   treatment failure, 51f
herd immunity, 94
herpes simplex infection, 51–54
   aetiology, 52
   coldsore, 53, 53f
   eczema herpeticum, 35, 36f
   epidemiology, 51–52
   prevention, 53–54
   stages, 51, 52f
   treatment, 54
herpes simplex virus (HSV)
   aciclovir effects, 54
   infection *see* herpes simplex infection
   type-1, 53
   type-2, 53
histamine
   H1-receptor antagonists in pruritus, 84
   urticaria aetiology, 100
histiocytoma *see* dermatofibroma (histiocytoma)
HIV infection/AIDS
   molluscum contagiosum, 70
   seborrhoeic eczema, 43
hormones
   acne aetiology, 8–9
   acne treatment, 13
   Addison's disease, 25
   pruritus, 83f
house dust mite, atopic eczema, 34
human papilloma virus (HPV), 113
   see also warts (viral)

hydroa vacciniforme, 78
hydrocortisone, 133t
hydrocortisone butyrate, 134t
hydroxychloroquine, discoid lupus erythematosus, 32
hygiene hypothesis, 34
hyperpigmentation, post-inflammatory, 61
hypopigmentation *see* vitiligo

I

ichthammol, 134t
ichthyosiform erythrodermas, 54
ichthyosis, 35, 54–55, 55f
   aetiology, 55
   epidemiology, 54
   treatment, 55
   X-linked, 54–55, 56f
ichthyosis vulgaris, 54, 55, 56f
imidazole antifungals, 27
imiquimod
   actinic keratosis, 16f, 17f
   molluscum contagiosum, 71
   warts, 118
immune factors
   atopic eczema, 33–34
   lichen planus, 59–60
   mast cells, 99, 100, 104
   see also allergy/allergens
immunofluorescence, discoid lupus erythematosus, 32
immunoglobulin E (IgE), atopic eczema, 33–34
immunosuppressive drugs, eczema, 37f
impetigo, 56–57, 57f
   treatment, 58
   types, 57f
infections
   bacterial *see* bacterial infections
   dermatophyte *see* dermatophyte infections
   eczema/dermatitis, 36–37
   fungal *see* fungal infections
   scabies, 96
   viral *see* viral infection
   see also specific infections
intradermal injections, triamcinolone, 19
isotretinoin, 13–14, 140t, 141t
   dosage and monitoring, 14
   relapse rates, 15

side-effects, 14, 14f
Isotrex, 140t
Isotrexin, 140t
itching *see* pruritus
itraconazole, 148t
   pityriasis versicolor, 80
   seborrhoeic eczema, 44
ivermectin, scabies, 96

K

keratinization, altered patten in acne,
   9
keratoacanthoma, 58–59, 58f
ketoconazole, 146t, 148t
Köbner phenomenon, 114

L

Lamisil, 147t, 148t
lanolin, 40f
leg ulcers
   non-venous, 109f
   venous, 108–111, 108f
   see also venous ulcers
lentigo maligna, 66
lesions
   artefactual, 19, 20f, 21f
   facial, basal cell carcinoma, 22
   lupus erythematosus, 31f
   mucous membrane, lichen planus,
      60
   typical acne lesions, 8f, 9f
leucocytoclastic vasculitis, 105, 106f,
   107f
lice, head *see* head lice
lichen planopilaris, 60
lichen planus, 59–62, 60f
   aetiology, 59–60
   autoimmune disease and, 59
   diagnosis, 60
   drug-induced, 60, 123–124cs,
      123f, 124f
   epidemiology, 59
   lesions, 61
   nails, 60–61
   photosensitivity, 78
   post-inflammatory hyperpigmen-
      tation, 61
   prevention, 61
   treatment, 62
   variants, 61f
lichen simplex, 62–63
   features, 62

treatment, 63, 63f
light *see* ultraviolet (UV) radiation
lip licking, 20f
liquid nitrogen, actinic keratosis, 16f,
   17f
Locoid, 134t
Lotriderm, 128t
lupus erythematosus, 31
   discoid *see* discoid lupus erythe-
      matosus
   photosensitivity, 78
   vasculitis, 106f
Lyclear Creme Rinse, 150t
Lyclear Dermal Cream, 150t
lymphoma, ichthyosis, 55

M

Malathion, 50, 150t
   scabies, 96
malignancy
   causing pruritus, 83f
   warts, 115
   see also specific cancers
malignant melanoma, 66–69
   acral, 67
   aetiology, 66
   atypical mole syndrome,
      121–122cs, 121f, 122f
   Breslow thickness *vs.* survival,
      68–69, 68f
   diagnosis, 66, 67–68, 68f
   epidemiology, 66
   growth pattern, 66
   lentigo maligna (melanoma), 66
   nodular, 67, 67f
   prevention, 69
   superficial spreading, 67, 67f
   treatment, 69
   see also melanocytic naevi
mast cells
   stabilizing drugs, 104
   urticaria, 99, 100
Maxtrex, 138t
melanocytes, vitiligo, 111
melanocytic naevi, 64–65
   atypical mole syndrome,
      121–122cs, 121f, 122f
   diagnosis, 65
   epidemiology, 64–65
   malignant melanoma risk factor,
      66
   treatment, 65

variants, 64f
melanoma *see* malignant melanoma
metabolic disorders, pruritus, 83f
methotrexate, 138t
    psoriasis, 89f
Metrogel, 145t
metronidazole, 145t
    rosacea, 92
Metrosa, 145t
Metrotop, 145t
miconazole, 133t, 146t
Microsporum canis, 28f
miliaria rubra (prickly heat), 77
Minocin, 142t
minocycline, 13, 142t
minoxidil, 144t
mizolastine, urticaria, 104
moccasin foot, 29f
Modrasone, 128t
moles *see* melanocytic naevi
molluscum contagiosum, 69–72, 70f
    aetiology, 70
    diagnosis, 71
    epidemiology, 70
    prevention, 71
    treatment, 71–72
    types, 71f
mometasone furoate, 134t
mucocutaneous candidiasis, 25, 25f
mucous membrane lesions, lichen
    planus, 60
mupirocin, 145t
    treatment, 58

N

naevi, 64–65, 64f
    see also melanocytic naevi
nails
    artefactual skin disease, 20f
    lichen planus, 60–61
    psoriasis, 88
    tinea infection, 30f
necrotizing fasciitis, 48
neomycin, 129t, 130t, 132t
    impetigo treatment, 58
Neoral, 138t
Neotigason, 138t
Nerisone, 131t
neurotic excoriations, 20f
Nicam, 140t
nickel, contact dermatitis, 40f
nicotinamide, 140t

nits, 50
    see also head lice
Nizoral, 146t, 148t
nodular melanoma, 67
nodules
    ear, painful, 72, 73f
    malignant melanoma, 67, 67f
    scabies, 93f
    vasculitis, 105
Noritate, 145t
NSAID-induced lichen planus,
    123–124cs, 123f, 124f
Nystan, 146t
nystatin, 130t, 133t, 146t

O

Occlusal, 143t
occupational dermatitis, 39, 39f
onycholysis, 88
oral lichen planus, 60, 124f
    treatment, 62
oxytetracycline, 12–13, 130t, 142t

P

PanOxyl, 139t
paronychia, 25f
patch testing
    contact dermatitis, 41
    urticaria, 102, 103
pediculicides, 50–51
pellagra, 77
pemphigoid, 73–75, 73f
    aetiology, 74
    diagnosis, 74
    differential diagnosis, 74f
    epidemiology, 73–74
    treatment, 74–75
penciclovir, 148t
    herpes simplex, 54
penicillin, erysipelas, 48
permethrin, 150t
    scabies, 96
perniosis (chilblains), 105
pevaryl, 146t
phenothrin, 150t
phenylenediamines, 40f
photochemotherapy, eczema, 37f
photodynamic therapy, actinic kerato-
    sis, 16f, 17f
photosensitivity, 75–79
    causes, 76f
    disorders exacerbated by light,

78–79
hydroa vacciniforme, 78
pellagra, 77
polymorphic light eruption, 77–78, 78f
porphyria, 77
solar urticaria, 77
sunburn, 75–76, 76f
pilosebaceous follicles, acne, 9
pimecrolimus, 135t
eczema/dermatitis, 37f, 44
seborrhoeic eczema, 44
pityriasis versicolor, 79–80
aetiology, 79
diagnosis, 79
treatment, 79–80
Pityrosporum, 43
plane wart, 118
plant antigens, 40f
plantar warts, 114, 118
podophyllotoxin, 118
pollen, atopic eczema, 34
polyarteritis nodosa, 106f
polycystic ovarian syndrome, acne, 9
polymorphic light eruption, 77–78, 78f
prevention, 78
Polytar Emollient, 136t
porphyria, 77
porphyria cutanea tarda, 77
post-inflammatory hyperpigmentation, 61
pox virus, 70
prednisolone, lichen planus, 62
pregnancy, scabies, 96
prickly heat (miliaria rubra), 77
Prioderm, 150t
Propecia, 144t
Propionibacterium acnes, 9
Protopic, 135t
pruritogens, 81f
pruritus, 81–84
aetiology, 81
definition, 81
diagnosis, 81
diagnostic decisions, 82f
pathways involved, 80f
pruritogens, 81f
treatment, 82–84, 83f
psoriasis, 84–88, 86f, 119–120cs, 120f
aetiology, 85
arthropathic, 87, 88f
chronic of palms and soles, 87
classical plaque, 85, 87f
diagnosis, 85–88
epidemiology, 84
flexural, 86
guttate, 85–86
histology, 84f
nail changes, 88
photosensitivity, 78
prevention, 88
pustular, 86–87
treatment, 88, 89f
unstable/erthrodermic, 87
variants, 85f
von Zumbusch, 87
psychological factors
acne treatment, 14
artefactual skin disease, 19, 20f, 21f
imaginary lice, 50
rosacea, 92
pustular psoriasis, 86–87
PUVA therapy
polymorphic light eruption, 78
psoriasis, 89f
squamous cell carcinoma and, 98
vitiligo, 112
pyogenic granuloma, 90–91, 90f

Q
Quellada M, 150t

R
radioallergosorbent (RAST) testing, urticaria, 102, 103
radiotherapy
basal cell carcinoma, 23
squamous cell carcinoma, 99
Regaine, 144t
Retin-A, 140t
retinoic acid, actinic keratosis, 16f, 17f
retinoid, 13f
Retinova, 140t, 144t
rhinophyma, rosacea, 91f, 92
ringworm infection, 27f, 28f
Roaccutane, 141t
rosacea, 91–93, 91f
acne vs., 10
aetiology, 91–92
complications, 92
epidemiology, 91

factors exaggerating, 92f
photosensitivity, 78
treatment, 92–93
Rozex, 145t
rubber chemicals, 40f

S
Salactol, 143t
Salatac, 143t
salicylic acid, 128t, 129t, 130t, 143t
psoriasis, 89f
seborrhoeic eczema, 44
warts (viral), 116, 116f, 118
Sarcoptes scabiei, 94
see also scabies
scabies, 93–96
aetiology, 94–95
crusted (Norwegian), 95
diagnosis, 95
differential diagnosis, 94f
epidemiology, 94
future developments, 96
infections, 96
prevention, 95
scrotal nodules, 93f
treatment, 95–96
scalp
alopecia, 19f
see also alopecia areata
lice *see* head lice
ringworm, 28f
scaly patches, actinic keratosis, 15–16
scarring
acne, 8
dermatofibroma (histiocytoma),
25–27
scratching, lichen simplex, 62, 63
scrotal nodules, scabies, 93f
seborrhoeic eczema, 34f, 43–44, 43f,
79
infantile, 43
treatment, 44
seborrhoeic keratosis, 97–98, 97f
diagnosis, 97
treatment, 98
sebum
acne, 8–9
isotretinoin, 13
sexually transmitted diseases
HSV-2 infections, 53
molluscum contagiosum, 70
warts, 118

Silkis, 136t
silver nitrate, 143t
Skinoren, 139t
soap substitutes, 127f
Solaraze, 143t
spitz naevus, 64f
Sporanox, 148t
squamous cell carcinoma, 98–99, 99f
actinic keratosis *vs.*, 16
aetiology, 98
invasive, 23–24
prevention, 99
in situ (Bowen's disease), 23–24,
24f
treatment, 99
staphylococcal infection
eczema/dermatitis, 36–37
impetigo, 57f
Staphylococcus aureus, 36–37
stasis eczema *see* varicose (stasis)
eczema
steroids *see* corticosteroids
steroid sulphatase deficiency, 55
Stiedex, 130t
Stiemycin, 139t
streptococcal infection
erysipelas, 46, 46f
impetigo, 57f
suicide, isotretinoin, 14
sulconazole, 147t
sun exposure/sunburn, 75–76, 77
actinic keratosis, 15
basal cell carcinoma, 22
discoid lupus erythematosus, 31
keratoacanthoma, 58f
malignant melanoma, 66
prevention, 77
squamous cell carcinoma, 99
susceptibility of skin types, 76f
treatment, 77
see also ultraviolet (UV) radiation
swimming pools, molluscum contagiosum, 69, 70, 71
Synalar, 132t
systemic lupus erythematosus, photosensitivity, 78
systemic steroids, alopecia areata, 19

T
tacalcitol, 137t
tacrolimus, 135t
eczema/dermatitis, 37f

seborrhoeic eczema, 44
tar
    coal, 136t
    eczema, 37f
    psoriasis, 89f
taraotene, 137t
teratogenicity, isotretinoin, 14
terbinafine, 27, 147t, 148t
tetracyclines, 12–13, 142t
Timodine, 133t
tinea pedis, 28
    contact dermatitis, 125–126cs,
    125f, 126f
    diagnosis and management, 29f
topical steroids
    alopecia areata, 18–19
    discoid lupus erythematosus, 32
    lichen planus, 62
    vitiligo, 112
topical treatments
    acne, 11, 12f
    actinic keratosis, 16f, 17f
    alopecia areata, 18–19
    dermatophytes, 28f, 29, 29f, 30f
    molluscum contagiosum, 71
    steroids *see* topical steroids
    see also specific treatments
Topicycline, 139t
tretinoin, 140t, 144t
triamcinolone, intradermal injections,
    19
Trichophyton rubrum, 29f
Trichophyton schoenleinii, 28f
Trichophyton tonsurans, 28f
Trichophyton verrucosum, 28f
'tri-chrome' vitiligo, 112
trimethoprim, 13
Trimovate, 130t

U

ulcers
    leg *see* leg ulcers
    non-venous, 109f
    venous *see* venous ulcers
ultraviolet B (UVB) radiation
    psoriasis, 89f
    squamous cell carcinoma, 98
    sunburn, 75
ultraviolet (UV) radiation
    basal cell carcinoma, 22
    Bowen's disease, 23
    disorders exacerbated by, 78–79

melanoma, 69
photosensitivity *see* photosensitiv-
    ity
    as treatment *see* PUVA therapy
    see also sun exposure/sunburn
urea, 133t
urticaria, 99–105
    causes, 102f, 103f
    classifications, 101f
    diagnosis, 100–103
    differential diagnosis, 102
    epidemiology, 100
    treatment, 103–105, 104
    types, 102–103
urticarial vasculitis, 102, 105, 106f

V

valaciclovir, 149t
    herpes simplex, 54
Valtrex, 149t
varicose (stasis) eczema, 44–46
    diagnosis, 45, 45f
    epidemiology, 44
    treatment, 45–46
vasculitis, 105–106
    aetiology, 105
    classification, 106f
    clinical features, 107f
    diagnosis, 106
    epidemiology, 105
    leucocytoclastic, 105, 106f, 107f
    nodular, 105
    treatment, 106
    urticarial, 105, 106f
Vectavir, 148t
venous hypertension, features,
    108–109
venous insufficiency, varicose (stasis)
    eczema, 45
venous ulcers, 108–111
    aetiology, 108–109
    compression, 111
    diagnosis, 109
    prevention, 109
    treatment, 109–110
Veracur, 142t
verruca, 113f
Verrugon, 143t
Vibramycin, 141t
viral infection
    HIV infection/AIDS, 43, 70
    HSV *see* herpes simplex infection

warts *see* warts (viral)
vitamin A analogues, psoriasis, 89f
vitamin D analogues, psoriasis, 89f
vitiligo, 111–113, 112f
    aetiology, 111
    diagnosis, 111–112
    epidemiology, 111
    prevention, 112
    treatment, 112–113
von Zumbusch psoriasis, 87

W

warts (viral), 113–118, 113f, 114f
    aetiology, 114
    clinical pattern and HPV type,
    114f
    diagnosis, 114–115
    differential diagnosis, 115f
    epidemiology, 113–114
    genital (HSV-2 infection), 53–54
    malignancy and, 115
    prevention, 115

    specialist therapy, 118f
    treatment, 115–118, 116–118f
    see also specific types
websites, 152–157
Wegener's granulomatosis, 106f
wet-wrapping, eczema, 36
wood antigens, 40f

X

Xepin, 134t
xerosis, 35
X-linked ichthyosis, 54–55, 56f

Y

yeast infections, 79–80
    seborrhoeic eczema, 43

Z

Zineryt, 139t
Zorac, 137t
Zovirax, 148t, 149t